LAW AND PSYCHIATRY II

Proceedings of the Second International Symposium
Held at the Clarke Institute of Psychiatry,
Toronto, Canada, February 1978

LAW AND PSYCHIATRY II

Proceedings of the Second International Symposium
Held at the Clarke Institute of Psychiatry,
Toronto, Canada, February 1978

David N. Weisstub
Editor
Visiting Professor of Psychiatry,
Clarke Institute of Psychiatry, University of Toronto,
and Professor of Law, Osgoode Hall Law School of
York University, Toronto, Canada

Pergamon Press

NEW YORK • OXFORD • TORONTO • SYDNEY • FRANKFURT • PARIS

Pergamon Press Offices:

U.S.A.	Pergamon Press, Inc., Maxwell House, Fairview Park, Elmsford, New York 10523, U.S.A.
U.K.	Pergamon Press Ltd., Headington Hill Hall, Oxford OX3 0BW, England
CANADA	Pergamon of Canada, Ltd., 150 Consumers Road, Willowdale, Ontario M2J 1P9, Canada
AUSTRALIA	Pergamon Press (Aust) Pty. Ltd., P. O. Box 544, Potts Point, New South Wales 2011, Australia
FRANCE	Pergamon Press SARL, 24 rue des Ecoles, 75240 Paris, Cedex 05, France
FEDERAL REPUBLIC OF GERMANY	Pergamon Press GmbH, 6242 Kronberg/Taunus, Pferdstrasse 1, West Germany

Library of Congress Cataloging in Publication Data

International Symposium in Law and Psychiatry, 2d,
    Clarke Institute of Psychiatry, 1978.
    Law and Psychiatry II.

    1. Mental health laws--Congresses. 2. Forensic
psychiatry--Congresses. 3. Psychology, Forensic--
Congresses.   I. Weisstub, David, 1944-   II. Title.
K3608.A55I57 1978   344.04'4   78-26644
ISBN 0-08-023901-3

Printed in the United States of America

CONTENTS

Preface

The Pendulum Swings from Society to the Individual

The relationship between law and psychiatry has a history of several millennia, dating back at least to ancient Egyptian and Biblical times when the word "psychiatrist" did not exist. Indeed, from the beginnings of recorded history there is evidence that social policy was formulated to deal with the impact of states of mind upon the behavior of individuals. Yet although lawyers, mental health professionals and the public at large usually have found this a topic of fascination, it is also true that until quite recently issues of forensic psychiatry have been at the periphery of attention of practicing professionals, except of course for the specialists in the field itself.

Today, however, for most psychiatrists and many psychologists and lawyers certain issues have moved from the back chapters of textbooks to the forefront of daily attention, particularly issues related to revisions of mental health legislation and to redefinitions of patients' rights, the limits of professional obligation and authority, and the principles of management of socially dissident or dangerous behavior. These issues touch not only on the patterns of practice of these professionals but at times also on their actual roles and identity.

These are the very issues addressed by the conference which provided the content of this volume. The Second International Symposium on Law and Psychiatry, convened by the Clarke Institute of Psychiatry and Osgoode Hall Law School, like its predecessor of the year before,[1] brought together in Toronto an international, multidisciplinary group of academics and practitioners who are eminently qualified to consider these problems. Even more broadly than its predecessor this second symposium examined some current manifestations of the age-old dialectic between advocates of the rights of the individual and of the rights of his society. In this debate at various periods in history, one side or the other has had the initiative. There are many reasons for believing that during the past two decades a shift back in favor of the individual has started after at least half a century during which the needs of society were seen as paramount. I refer here to the replacement of the liberal, humanitarian ideals of the 19th century, which followed the American and French revolutions, by the materialistic view of man as servant of the collectivity (the nation, the state, the proletariat, etc.) which has swept much of the world in this century.

With reference to the position of society's unfortunates — the neglected child, the mentally ill, the social misfit or deviant — the need for protection of society and for its protective authority over the individual (parens patriae) has held sway during this period. In part this has been fueled by the optimism engendered by advances in understanding biological and psychodynamic determinants of motivation and behavior. At least since the Freudian revolution at the

---

[1] D. N. Weisstub, ed., *Law and Psychiatry* (New York: Pergamon Press, 1978).

turn of the century (and in part as a result of it) the belief grew that much
social pathology as well as frank psychiatric disorder can be eliminated if these
determining factors are controlled. Thus the state via the legal process has been
authorized increasingly to act on behalf of its citizens who are mentally ill, psy-
chologically impaired or considered at risk for such impairment. Psychiatrists
have been both catalysts and agents of this process. We have permitted, and at
times encouraged, a massive extension of our societal mandate far beyond its
traditional clinical roots.[2] The countercurrent is now swirling strongly to the
point of threatening to upset many professionals sailing along on traditional
courses. The shift of focus from the needs of society and its agents to the rights
of the individual is readily apparent at the intersection of law and psychiatry. A
reading of the papers in this volume and the discussion they provoked reflects
this shift, although I do not believe that the convenors of the symposium originally had this specific theme in mind.

In his paper, "The Many-Headed Psychiatrist," Zeegers describes the many
hats that we, Hydra-like, attempt to wear today. Some of these are traditional,
appropriate and necessary for our primary role of scientifically informed healers of disordered patients; some are quite anachronistic and most of us would
gladly discard them; some are accepted by our fellow professionals and by the
public, while others are now in dispute. Zeegers suggests a limitation on the
number of heads and hats and he offers an idealistic, humanistic direction for
the field.

Robitscher in "The Limits of Psychiatric Authority" takes this further. His
closely reasoned paper, in the tradition of Szasz, Laing, Torrey and other critics-
from-within, illuminates the ethical, legal and professional dilemmas of the
failure of the psychiatric profession itself to delineate the limits of its authority.
In discussing Zeeger's paper, Slovenko goes further still in this regard.

The same spirit of support for the individual and his family in the face of a
benevolent but at times crudely destructive paternalistic state is evident in the
paper by Goldstein, "Psychoanalysis and a Jurisprudence of Child Placement."
Summarizing a theme which he develops further with Anna Freud and Albert
Solnit in *Beyond the Best Interests of the Child* and the forthcoming *Before
the Best Interests of the Child,* Goldstein points to the limited capacity of the
state (in this case acting through Family Court judges, Children's Aid Societies,
etc.) to act constructively on behalf of the child at risk. Consequently he argues:
"The Law must hold in check the rescue phantasies of those it empowers to intrude [on family relationships on behalf of a child]."

---

[2] Consider, for example, a strong but not atypical statement advocating such extension only a decade
ago: "My point is that the knowledge and experience of the psychiatrist should enter into the counsels of
men where and when the patterns, symptoms, and values of our new existence are under consideration.
More specifically, I intend that psychiatry in its varied gnostic segments, normal, developmental, prophy-
lactic, diagnostic and therapeutic, should be available to serve teacher, statesman, manager, engineer,
minister, politician, legislator and the like. It should be available to serve, not on 'beck and call,' but as
much on the initiative of the psychiatrist as on those to be served. I propose for psychiatry a more effective role in the shaping of civilization so that civilization might prove less baneful to mankind." I. Gald-
ston, "Civilization and its Discontents," in Aldwyn B. Stokes, ed., *Psychiatry in Transition 1966-1967*
(Toronto: University of Toronto Press, 1967), p. 136.

Perhaps the most direct expression of the society-to-individual shift is the current patients' rights movement in the United States. Mental health advocates in a very few years have won an astonishing series of major judicial decisions which have defined and extended a number of patient rights. These are discussed most authoritatively by Wald and Friedman, which is not surprising since they are very close indeed to the action. That simply obtaining judicial affirmation of rights does not solve highly complex social problems is at once clear from their well balanced paper. There are rights which can conflict (e.g., at times the right to treatment needs to be weighed against the right to liberty). There is the recent tendency of courts actively to usurp the authority of legislatures in setting public policy and priorities. There is also at times tension between legal controls and treatment goals. But the thrust of the shift is toward the individual.

Two papers in this volume deal with specific groups of people whose identity as psychiatric patients has been at times affirmed and at times denied. Jensen makes an interesting conceptual contribution to the concept of *psychopathy* which he believes to be a legitimate entity, in contrast to the *psychopath,* whom he sees as a victim of societal labeling which compounds a defect in the capacity for interpersonal morality. But the interesting point, with respect to the theme which I am considering here, is that Jensen stresses the overriding need to understand the experience of the individual though he works in a setting (Herstedvester) which is a maximum security prison clearly intended to protect society from the inmates.

Finally, with respect to revision of mental health legislation, Dabrowski reports that Poland in its new draft proposal joins several jurisdictions in Western Europe and North America which have moved to extend the rights of psychiatric patients. Although commentators on this paper criticize the Polish draft with respect to alleged ambiguities, mechanisms and safeguards (i.e., whether the legislation as it will be applied will advance the stated aims), there is no mistaking these aims as they are proclaimed.

This volume then is timely as a reflection of the Zeitgeist, emphasizing the shift from the needs of society to the protection of the rights of the individual. What is more, it contains some excellent papers, contributions which can have a salutary organizing influence on the thought of various professionals interested in the interaction of law and psychiatry.

Frederick H. Lowy
Director and Psychiatrist-in-Chief
Clarke Institute of Psychiatry

Professor and Chairman
Department of Psychiatry
University of Toronto

Introduction

These proceedings are the result of a three-day conference which took place under the auspices of the Clarke Institute of Psychiatry of the University of Toronto, and Osgoode Hall Law School of York University. The opening lecture was delivered by Professor Joseph Goldstein of Yale Law School on a subject for which he has gained an international reputation: the role of counsel for children in family law. This session was moderated by Mr. Justice Arthur Martin of the Court of Appeal for Ontario. The conference participants included delegates from across Canada, as well as from foreign jurisdictions, who brought to the discussions their different theoretical, organizational and practical perspectives.

The paper by Professor Dabrowski is of particular interest. It outlines the principal elements of a new Mental Health Act which is now at the final stages of review and implementation in Poland. This Act is the distillation of five years work by a committee of experts, and may represent a model for other Eastern European countries in drafting legislative revisions. The commentaries following the Dabrowski address are comparative, and emphasize English and American developments in mental health legislation.

Patricia M. Wald and Paul R. Friedman summarize the seminal themes in the evolution of an American jurisprudence on mental health law. The United States has seen in the past decade a sudden emergence of litigation and reform projects affecting almost every aspect of mental health practice. Indeed, many of the significant changes are the direct result of the collaborative work of Wald and Friedman through the Mental Health Law Project in Washington, D.C. Some of the United States breakthroughs have been controversial, and in the context of a primarily Canadian audience, it was instructive to consider the responses of members of the Department of Justice and the judiciary who in their work assess the value of American trends for Canada.

Dr. Ole Jensen's essay on the "Mask of Psychopathy," through the use of case examples, points out the centrality of socio-cultural variables to the designation of psychopathy. Dr. Roosenburg, who replies to Jensen, speaks from a unique familiarity with psychopathy. Many persons continue to regard Dr. Roosenburg as the leading authority on psychopathy in Western Europe. In his comments, Dr. Cormier of McGill University adds a subtle philosophical understanding of the concept.

The forum was honored by the lecture of Dr. Jonas Robitscher on the subject of the limits of psychiatric authority. Dr. Robitscher elaborates here on the themes contained in his Isaac Ray Lectures of 1976. His remarks are cause for extensive reflection as they touch upon basic problems relating to the roles and functions of professional psychiatry.

Dr. Michael Zeegers, in "The Many Headed Psychiatrist," analyzes the many roles which the psychiatrist can assume and discusses the dangers he perceives in the adoption of some of these functions. Professor Cyril Greenland analyzes the social policy issues involved in the prediction of "dangerousness." His lecture represents a stocktaking of current data and invites in-depth research to afford proper answers to balancing individual liberty against social protection.

The conference was co-organized by Dr. R. E. Turner, and I wish to record my thanks to him for his conscientious endeavors. Ms. Linda Davey has proven an invaluable editorial collaborator in the final preparation of these proceedings. We are all deeply indebted to the sponsorship of the Canadian Department of Justice and the Department of National Health and Welfare who have taken seriously our attempts to foster international multidisciplinary exchanges. The Ontario Law Foundation, through a generous grant, has made possible the publication of this volume.

David N. Weisstub
Editor

Psychoanalysis and a Jurisprudence of Child Placement — with Special Emphasis on the Role of Legal Counsel for Children

Joseph Goldstein*

The law of child placement and the ways in which that jurisprudence may be illumined by psychoanalytic notions about healthy growth and development is what I wish to discuss.

As a lawyer who happens to be a Psychoanalyst (not a psychoanalyst who happens to be a lawyer), I propose to develop a framework for determining what events or circumstances in the life of a child should justify coercive intervention by the state on the private ordering of that child's relationship with his parents. I propose to construct a model for evaluating state intrusions on the essence of family life, for identifying and assessing the ways in which the law is invoked to protect, to shatter and to create opportunities for children and their parents to "feel at home,"[1] to "be secure in their persons [and in their] houses."[2]

In our book, *Beyond the Best Interests of the Child,* Anna Freud, Albert J. Solnit and I were primarily concerned with problems confronting children about to be or already caught up in the legal process. On the basis of common sense, reenforced by psychoanalytic knowledge, we sought to establish, in accord with the law's overall commitment to serving the child's best interests, guidelines for determining the least detrimental procedure for making his placement.

In *Beyond the Best Interests of the Child,* we did not ask when and why a child's placement ought to become a matter of state concern. We did not consider what must happen to or in the life of a child *before* the state should be allowed to invoke the best interests standard. We did not critically examine the state's justifications for placing a family under scrutiny. We did not consider, for example, whether the divorce of parents or the separation of unmarried parents should in themselves be sufficient grounds for state intervention to decide, not only who should have custody of their children, but also to continually monitor and determine when, if ever, the newly established legal relationships should be changed. Nor did we go much beyond questioning (to take one

---

*Walton Hale Hamilton Professor of Law, Science and Social Policy, Yale University Law School, New Haven, Connecticut 06520; and Professor, Yale University Child Study Center.

[1] Talk by James Anthony in New Haven, Connecticut (April 9, 1977).
[2] U.S. Const., amend. IV (1791).

other example) the vague, imprecise and subjective criteria of neglect statutes which empower the state to scrutinize and supervene an individual parent's authority. The question which underlies these examples, and one aspect of which this article will begin to address, is: What ought to have to be established *before* a particular child's interest becomes a matter for the law rather than for his parents to decide?

In order to clarify the scope of such an inquiry and to place in context the grounds for state intervention which might emerge as substitutes for those now provided in abuse, delinquency, divorce and neglect law, it becomes necessary to *identify the values and presumptions* which underlie our jurisprudence of child placement and to *make visible the separate questions* answered, though not necessarily consciously posed, by legislator, judge and administrator in their child placement decisions.

Minimum State Intervention Versus Making the Child's Interests Paramount

Without explicitly defining "family," the law assumes that "family" is an essential component of the "good" society and that "family," like law, is one of the basic processes for the control of human behavior. In a work session on our forthcoming book which will be entitled, *Before the Best Interests of the Child,* Anna Freud observed:

> A privilege of childhood is to be sheltered from direct contact with the law and to have society's and the state's demands and prohibitions filtered by way of the parent's personalities. The parents thus not only represent the law to the child, but are also his representatives before the law.

Indeed, the law of child placement may be perceived as a response to the "success" or "failure" of parents in fulfilling their task of nourishing in their children the internal mechanisms of control sufficient for each one, upon becoming an adult, to be a law unto himself, but not above the law. Indeed, in the eyes of the law, to be a *child* is to be at risk, dependent and without capacity or authority to decide free of parental control what is "best" for oneself. To be an *adult* is to be perceived in law as free to take risks, as independent and with the capacity and authority to decide to do what is "best" for oneself without regard to parental wishes. Therefore, to be an *adult who is parent* is to be presumed by law to have the capacity, authority and responsibility to determine and to do what is "good" for one's children, what is "best" for the entire family. It thus becomes the function of the law to protect family privacy as a means of safeguarding parental autonomy in childrearing as well as each child's entitlement to autonomous parents who wish to be responsible for the child's care.

Family privacy, parental autonomy and the child's entitlement to autonomous parents together give content to the notion of "family integrity" as a liberty interest which is worthy of protection from state interference.[3] We use

---

[3] Stanley v. Illinois, 405 U.S. 645, 657 (1972).

the encompassing phrase "family integrity," rather than family autonomy," to highlight that the autonomy to be protected by law lies with the adults, who as parents, are responsible for determining the ambit of their own children's autonomy. As the late Mr. Justice Harlan of the United States Supreme Court declared, "The home derives its preeminence as the seat of family life. And the integrity of that life is something so fundamental that it has been found to draw to its protection the principles of more than one explicitly granted constitutional right."[4] Further, at least two separate parent-child relationships have deserved recognition and protection from interruption by the state. One, often thought to be the only one, is the entitlement of natural parents and their children to each other — an interest which rests on the fact of biological reproduction and arises when a child is born — an interest which may be lost or destroyed in a psychological, a real, sense unless it is continuously nurtured. The other protected interest, one not yet so firmly established as the biological but just as worthy of protection from coercive intrusion by the state, is in the psychological parent-child relationship, the "familial bonds" which develop with their long term caretakers without regard to biological ties.[5] John Locke recognized this more than three centuries ago, long before psychoanalysis but long after man began to think about the nature and needs of man, when he wrote:

> Nay, this [paternal] *power* so little belongs to the father by any peculiar right of nature, but only as he is guardian of his children, that when he quits his care of them, he loses his power over them, which goes along with their nourishment and education, to which it is inseparably annexed, and it belongs as much to the *foster-father* of an exposed child, as to the natural father or another; so little power does the bare *act of begetting* give a man over his issue, if all his care ends there, and this be all the title he hath to the name and authority of a father.[6]

The liberty interest in family integrity and in the familial bond which underlies a policy of minimum state intervention on parent-child relationships needs no greater justification for each of us as citizens in a democracy than that it comports with our fundamental commitment to individual freedom and human dignity. But these rights to parental autonomy and family privacy correspond as well with common sense as with our understanding as psychoanalysts of the critical need every child has for continued and unbroken care within a com-

---

[4] Poe v. Ullman, 367 U.S. 497, 551 (1961) (Harlan, J. dissenting); Griswold v. Connecticut, 381 U.S. 479 (1965) (Harlan, J. concurring).

[5] Smith v. Organization of Foster Families, 431 U.S. 816 (1977). [T]he importance of the familial relationship, to the individuals involved and to society, stems from the emotional attachments that derive from the intimacy of daily association and from the role it plays in 'promot[ing] a way of life' through the instruction of children . . . as well as from the fact of blood relationship. No one would seriously dispute that a deeply loving and interdependent relationship between an adult and a child in his or her care may exist even in the absence of a blood relationship. At least where a child has been placed in foster care as an infant, has never known his natural parents, and has remained continuously for several years in the care of the same foster parents, it is natural that the foster family should hold the same place in the emotional life of the foster child, and fulfill the same socializing functions as a natural family. For this reason we cannot dismiss the foster family as a mere collection of unrelated individuals." Id. at 844–845.

[6] John Locke, *The Second Treatise of Government* (London; J. M. Dent & Sons, 1924) p. 147.

munity of concerned and intimately connected adults. No other animal is "sent into the world in a less finished state"[7] and is for so long a time after birth so helpless that its survival depends upon continuous nurture by adults. "This biological factor, then establishes the earliest situations of danger and creates *the need to be loved* which will accompany the child through the rest of its life."[8] It is that *need* which is generally best served when the reciprocal interests of children and parents in each other as members of a family are recognized and protected from interruption.

Court or agency intervention without regard to or over the objection of parents can only serve to undermine for children of any age ties which are vital to their sense of feeling at home and of becoming and being persons in their own right.[9] But to understand the danger of such state intrusion is not only to acknowledge how essential are autonomous parents to a child's well-being at each developmental stage, but is also to recognize the need for state intervention when parents fail. They may place their children at unwarranted risk. Family privacy may become a cover for exploiting the inherent inequality between adult and child. It may leave undetected the uncontrolled expression of the not uncommon unconscious, not to mention conscious, hatred some parents have for their children. That danger justifies state intervention in order to promote the goals of the very liberty interests in family integrity upon which it must intrude.

Yet to acknowledge that some parents may threaten the well-being of their children is not to suggest that state legislatures, courts or administrative agencies can always offer such children something better. By its intrusion the state may not only make a bad situation worse, it may turn a tolerable or good situa-

---

[7] Sigmund Freud, *Inhibitions, Symptoms, and Anxieties* (London: Hogarth Press, 1936) pp. 139–140. "The biological factor is the long period of time during which the young of the human species is in a condition of helplessness and dependence. Its intrauterine existence seems to be short in comparison with that of most animals, and it is sent into the world in a less finished state . . . Moreover, the dangers of the external world have a greater importance for it, so that the value of the object which can alone protect it against them and take the place of its former intra-uterine life is enormously enhanced. This biological factor, then, establishes the earliest situations of danger and creates *the need to be loved* which will accompany the child through the rest of its life." (Emphasis added).

Similarly, as long ago as 1840, Jeremy Bentham observed: "The feebleness of infancy demands a continual protection. Everything must be done for an imperfect being, which as yet does nothing for itself. The complete development of its physical powers takes many years; that of its intellectual faculties is still slower. At a certain age, it has already strength and passions,without experience enough to regulate them. Too sensitive to present impulses, too negligent of the future, such a being must be kept under an authority more immediate than that of the laws. . . ." (Jeremy Bentham, *Theory of Legislation,* ed. C. K. Ogden [London: Kegan Paul, Trench, Trubner & Co., 1931] p. 209.)

[8] Freud, *Inhibitions,* p. 140.

[9] Joseph Goldstein, Anna Freud, and Albert J. Solnit, *Beyond the Best Interests of the Child* (New York: Free Press, 1973) pp. 31–34. "The breaking or weakening of bonds has different, though almost always detrimental, consequences for children of different ages. For the very young, such events mean not only the painful rupture of emotional ties, but also the loss of many of the developmental achievements which are built on these ties such as impulse control, the rudiments of acceptable behavior and social adaptation. The more recently the achievement has been acquired, the more likely it is for a child to lose it – the lower his capacity for tolerating the severance of these fundamental relationships. For the adolescent it is critical to his sense of self and the integrity of his adulthood that the straining, even the breaking, of the bonds come exclusively from him and not be imposed either by parental abandonment or by force of law."

tion into a bad one. As *parens patriae* the state is too crude an instrument to become an adequate substitute for flesh and blood parents. The legal system has neither the resources nor the sensitivity to respond to a child's ever-changing needs and demands. It does not have the capacity to deal on an individual basis with the consequences of its decisions, nor to act with the deliberate speed required by a child's sense of time and essential to the child's well being. And, as Anna Freud observed in one of our work sessions: "The child does not have the capacity to respond to the rulings of an impersonal court as he responds to the demands of personal parental figures. The expectations, implicit and explicit, of parents become the child's own. However, the process by which a human being converts external commands and prohibitions into personal and internal ones does not function in the absence of the emotional ties which form the developmental base for them."

The laws of child placement must be revised to safeguard all families, poor and well-to-do, minority and majority, from state-sponsored interruptions of ongoing relationships by well-intentioned people who "know" what is "best" and who wish to impose their personal, even if professional, preferences on others. The law must hold in check the rescue fantasies of those it empowers to intrude. Thus, if the legislature is to give full recognition to a child's entitlement to a permanent family and the entitlement of parents to raise their children as they think best, it must reappraise the laws of child placement — particularly of abuse and neglect statutes — statutes which generally, vaguely and over-broadly, provide that a child "may be found 'neglected' who . . . is being denied proper care. . . ." In other words, *before* the best interests of the child standard can be invoked over the rights to parental autonomy, autonomous parents and family privacy, there is a need to determine what ought to have to be established and by what procedure.

As psychoanalysts and as citizens, we stated our preference in *Beyond the Best Interests of the Child* for a policy of minimum state intervention while developing guidelines that would accord with another preferred value about which we were equally explicit. We declared that once a child's custody had become the subject of a dispute over which the state had assumed jurisdiction, the law must make the child's needs paramount. Upon the belief that such children should be provided with an opportunity to be cared for by adults who are, or who are likely to become, their psychological parents, we proposed the following guidelines for determining a placement and the process of placement to accord with the best interests standard, or what we prefer to call the least detrimental available alternative standard:

1. Placement decisions should safeguard the child's need for continuity of relationships.
2. Placement decisions should reflect the child's, not the adult's, sense of time.
3. Child placement decisions must take into account the law's incapacity to supervise interpersonal relationships and the limits of knowledge to make long-range predictions.

With regard to this last guideline, some judges confuse their *authority* to do with their *capacity* to do.[10] They fail to realize that the *who* and *how* of custody are and must be separate. It is the *who*, which judges must and can decide. It is the *how* which is beyond any judge's competence. But judges often fail to see — what must be obvious once said — that the intricately delicate character of parent-child relationships place them beyond the judge's constructive reach, though not beyond their destructive reach.

Familial bonding is too complex and too vulnerable a process to be managed in advance or from the distance by so gross and impersonal an instrument as the law. In rejecting this simple, and unfortunately not sufficiently seductive guideline, the judges become oversimplifiers. They seduce themselves into believing that they can penetrate the blindfolds of justice to weigh and to assess the "amalgams of factors" which are beyond the competence of all other disciplines.

Were judges to follow the guidelines set forth in *Beyond the Best Interests of the Child,* they would restrict their activity to answering the one question that they really can and must answer; *who* shall have custody and not *how* nor *under what conditions* the custodians and child are to relate to one another and to others. But, like the well-intentioned, overprotective and often destructive parent who doesn't know when to let go, such judges decide not only who is to be parent, but also how the child is to be parented — for example, educated, medicated and visited.

The simple psychoanalytically informed guidelines of continuity, of a child's sense of time and of the limitations of law and knowledge, grew out of a recognition of how complex and vulnerable, not how simple or damage-proof, is the process of growing up. They recognize how vital it is to a child to be secure in the feeling that his "parents" are in charge and in control. Except for institutional placements and for temporary (truly short-term) foster care, judges, after deciding who shall have custody, must pull out decisively in the expectation that the adults selected can be relied upon to respond to their child's ever-changing day-to-day needs. Precisely because the human relationships in issue are complicated, courts and administrative agencies must have simple guidelines which, as each child is placed, will lead to an immediate and unequivocal restoration of family privacy, of parental autonomy and of non-intrusion. Simplicity is the ultimate sophistication in deciding a child's placement.

Fair Warning and Power Restraint: The Requirements of a Ground to Intrude

The law's response to "what should justify substituting the state's judgment for that of parents with regard to a particular child's care?" has taken two distinct forms. The first has been to set generally applicable and relatively precise limits on parental judgment concerning matters about which there is a clear societal consensus. For example, parents are not free to send their children into the labor market or to prevent them from attending school or from being immunized against certain contagious diseases. Such legislative enactments as those concerned with child labor, compulsory education and immunization are infringements upon parental autonomy. With relatively precise standards for

---

[10] Nanette Dembitz, "Beyond any Discipline's Competence," *Yale Law Journal* 83 (1974): 1304.

intervention, these statutes give all parents advance notice — fair warning — of what constitutes a breach of their child care responsibilities. The law thus restrains as well as grants the authority of court and administrative agency to breach the state's general commitment to family privacy and parental autonomy.

The second form which legislative responses take, and the one with which this article is concerned, sets relatively vague and imprecise limits on state authority to intrude and thus fails to provide fair warning. Those statutes concern child care matters about which there is no clear societal consensus. Though everyone may agree for example, that children ought not to be "neglected" or "abused" or that their "best interests" should be served, there is little agreement about the meaning of these terms. Legislative enactments, for example, which simply make "denial of proper care" the standard for investigating or determining "neglect," provide neither fair nor meaningful advance warning to parents nor adequate guidance for power restraint, for restricting the authority of the court or administrative agency to intervene.

This second form of legislation, unlike the first form, invests judges, agency and other state workers as *parens patriae,* with almost limitless discretion in areas generally under the exclusive control of parents. Such legislation is used to justify the ad hoc creation of standards of intervention in case-by-case determinations to investigate, to supervise and to supervene parental judgments. Its form invites the exploitation of parents and children by state officials. Acting in accord with their own personal childrearing preferences, they have discriminated against poor, minority, and other disfavored families.

To reduce unwarranted intrusions on family integrity, the laws of child placement must be recast to serve both a *fairwarning* function for parents and children and a *power restricting* function for state officials. Legislatures, therefore, must define prospectively and with greater precision than they currently do, their criteria for overcoming the strong presumptions in law that (a) parents have the right, the capacity, the authority and the obligation to care for and represent their children in accord with their own notions of child rearing, and that (b) children have the right to uninterrupted and permanent membership in a family with such parents.

But specificity of statutory language will never be enough to preclude unjustifiable invasions of family privacy. It is only a first and necessary condition for realizing the goals of fair warning and power restriction. Another necessary condition is that those who are empowered to intrude must understand, as well as share the bases for, a policy of minimum coercive state intervention.

A tradition, a culture in the administration of child placement laws which is sensitive to the notion of family integrity must be fostered. Further, we must recognize and seek to avoid the consequences of a fantasy too often unconsciously shared by those who define justifications and design procedures for intrusion. That fantasy is that only the most competent, most skilled and most sensitive lawyers, judges, doctors, social workers and other personnel will implement the laws of child placement. The reality is that there will always be a substantial number of persons in the process who do not meet that expectation. For that reason it is important to place a heavy evidentiary burden on those who are empowered to intrude as well as to establish procedures for intrusion which make highly visible the function, the nature, and the degree of intrusion that may be authorized at each point of decision.

In this context we seek to construct a framework for identifying and analyzing the process of decision.

Invocation, Adjudication and Disposition: Points of Decision

In order to locate the critical decisions in a child placement process guided by the doctrine of minimum state intervention, and in order to satisfy the requirements of fair warning and power restraint, it becomes necessary to focus briefly on three questions:

1. What should constitute *probable cause for inquiry* by the state into individual parent-child relationships?
2. What should constitute sufficient cause for the state to *modify* or *terminate* a parent-child relationship?
3. If there is sufficient cause for termination or modification, *can the state provide* the child with a *less detrimental placement?*

The three questions are seldom, if ever, confronted separately in child placement decisions. Yet each question is, in a real sense, answered in a continuous, though often muddled, flow of decisions by legislators, child care agency personnel and judges. Since those answers and the sequence in which they are rendered directly affect and often undermine society's commitment to family integrity, there is a need for a further refinement, to identify for separate consideration, the three critical stages of decision in the law of child placement which correspond to the three questions just posed. They are the stages of *invocation, adjudication* and *disposition.* Each state can be defined in terms of function and in terms of the degree and kind of coercive intrusion on family integrity that may be authorized.

Briefly, the function of the *invocation* stage is to determine whether a particular child's condition or circumstance justifies inquiry and the initiation of an action to overcome the presumption of parental autonomy. The function of the *adjudication* stage is to determine whether the child's condition or circumstance actually constitutes a statutory ground for supervening parental autonomy. The function of the *disposition* stage is to implement the adjudication. If no ground for supervention is established at adjudication, dismissal of the action is, of course, the disposition. If adjudication results in a finding that the parents have waived their autonomy, or that the presumption of autonomy has been overcome, the child then becomes for the first time a party to the proceedings and is entitled to legal representation, free of parental control. An adjudication which does not lead directly to a dismissal becomes a *suspended judgment* which cannot be acted upon until the court decides, following a hearing, what *disposition,* what placement, will provide the child with the least detrimental available alternative to accord with the child's best interests.

Supervening Parental Authority for Determining and Meeting the Legal Service Needs of their Children

Within the presumption of parental autonomy is the presumption that parents have, just as they do with regard to medical needs, the authority, duty and capacity to determine whether and how to meet their children's legal needs. Why and under what circumstances should that presumption be overcome and the state be authorized to appoint, without parental consent, legal counsel for a child? Parents or those selected by them are, or ought to be, the exclusive representatives of their children before the law. While the needs of the individual family members do not automatically coincide, the integrity of the family and the bonds that hold it together are so critical to the overall well-being of a child, that in general, they ought not to be severed by forcibly imposing an independent advocate between parent and child. Such interventions depose parents and deprive children of their privileged position of being sheltered by their parents from direct contact with the law.

Since the appointment of a child advocate without parental consent is a drastic alteration of the parent-child relationship it should generally follow — not precede — an adjudication that a ground has been established which justifies modifying or terminating the parent-child relationship. During the period of suspended judgment between adjudication and final disposition, a child requires party status and representation by legal counsel, independent of parents and child care agencies, to assure that the child's interests are represented and protected until the least detrimental available alternative has been chosen. At that point the "newly" designated parents should assume or resume responsibility, as autonomous parents, for determining all matters concerned with their child's care, including when and whether their child should have a lawyer and who that lawyer should be.

The confusion which underlies proposals supporting a child's right to legal counsel or an independent child advocate from the moment of invocation[11] may be clarified by examining a request for legal services made by Charlie Martin, a ten-year-old. He phoned me long distance and asked:

> Are you the lawyer who represents kids? I want you to help me. My parents are divorced. They're always fighting over visits with me and my sister Irene.

I told Charlie that before I could give him an answer I would have to know if the judge had already decided which of his parents had custody. He replied:

> My mother has custody. But why do you have to know that? I'm asking you to represent me.

I replied that since his mother had custody it was her responsibility to decide whether he needed the assistance of a lawyer and that if she decided that he needed one she would choose the lawyer she wanted for him. I would not represent him without his mother's consent, I said. He responded:

> I don't understand that, my mother may not want me to have a lawyer, and I want one.

I replied that what he wanted might not be what his mother thought best for him and that one of the reasons for having parents is to have someone to make such decisions for their children. I explained that just as parents were responsible for choosing their children's doctor and dentist and when to make appoint-

---

[11] IJA-ABA, *Standards Relating to Abuse and Neglect* (Cambridge: Ballinger, 1977) p. 96.

ments with them, it was also their responsibility to decide whether consulting a lawyer made sense. In Charlie's case I would not agree to his request unless his mother thought that he needed a lawyer and engaged me on his behalf. I asked Charlie if his mother knew about the phone call. He replied:

> Yes, she's right here. She'd like to talk to you.

Charlie's mother understood my position and after I explained that I preferred to do such work with a colleague who is a child analyst, she said that she wanted us to counsel Charlie and Irene concerning visits with their father. She said:

> I want the children to visit their father, I encourage them to do so. But, Charlie has "good reasons" for not wanting to observe the schedule established by the court. More important, my lawyers and those representing the children's father confuse the children with different explanations for why they must obey the court. Charlie keeps asking: "Why do we have to obey the court if Daddy doesn't? He can cancel visits." I want to clarify for Charlie and Irene what is going on.

I accepted her request on the understanding that we would counsel her children, advise her as to their needs — always making clear to them that she, as their custodial parent, had final say both with regard to accepting our advice and to our continuing to represent them. What we sought to accomplish on behalf of the two children in our negotiations with counsel for each of the parents and in testimony before the court was done with the consent and at the request of Mrs. Martin. We were guided by her wishes, by what she, as primary parent, ultimately determined would best serve the interests of her family.

Without going further into the relationship which developed between us and Charlie, Irene and their mother, I will describe only one event which occurred almost a year after we began serving them. Toward the close of a long winter holiday with his father (which his mother insisted he make), Charlie called us long distance and said:

> Call Mother. I don't want to go home. Tell her I'm staying with Daddy.

We told Charlie that we would try to reach his mother, that we would tell her about the call but that since she expected him to be home the next day he had to return unless she called to say it was "o.k." to stay. Charlie, obviously annoyed, said:

> You call her, tell her I'm not coming back. You're my lawyer you tell her what I want and get her to do it.

Again Charlie was reminded that his mother decided what he needed, that that was not always the same as what he wanted and that we did not tell his mother what she was to do. Despite our consistent efforts to respect parental autonomy, Charlie obviously thought that it was worth trying to maneuver us into a position which would undermine his mother's authority. When this failed, he returned home as scheduled.

What Charlie mistakenly sought to allocate to himself is the status of an adult. He tried to choose his counsel, instruct them with regard to his wishes and intentions, and, with their help fight his case with his parents or before the court. None of this is open to the child, unless, of course, his parents instruct counsel to abide by his wishes without regard to their specific references. At the very best, the child can expect to have his wishes taken into consideration by parents or their substitutes when they think that would be appropriate. In short, like Charlie, every child before the law finds himself in the position where the adult, father, mother, custodial parent, or state agency, "knows best" what is good for him and decides that regardless of the child's wishes.

I propose that the state restrict its *provision* of legal counsel for children to requests by parents who cannot obtain such assistance; and its *imposition* of such services without regard to parental wishes, to the disposition stage after an adjudication of at least one ground for modifying or terminating of parent-child relationships or, before such an adjudication during an emergency placement. Contrary to the current practice,[12] there would be no justification for the imposition of a child advocate at the invocation stage when a charge of neglect, abuse, or delinquency is made. To deprive parents at that point of their right to represent their child either through counsel of their own choice or without counsel and to appoint counsel for a child without parental consent would be to presume on the basis of an unproven — an unadjudicated — ground that parents are incompetent to serve the interests of their family and consequently the interests of their child. This would deprive a child, without due process, of his right to be represented by his parents before the law.[13]

On the other hand, not to appoint legal counsel for a child *following* an adjudication of a ground for modifying or terminating the child's relationship to the parents and *before* the *disposition* is determined would be to expose the child, uninsulated by an adult, to the state's authority. At that point (the disposition stage) — as well as during emergency placements prior to adjudication when a child is outside of parental care and control — a child requires a legal representative who will assure that the process of placement and the placement itself will make the child's interests paramount and provide the child with the least detrimental alternative.

The appointment of counsel may be perceived as a form of disposition, for a limited time and a limited purpose. The lawyer is to represent the child by gathering and providing the court with information relevant to determining the least harmful disposition. Court-imposed counsel is not a substitute nurturing parent. Nurture is to be provided by the caretakers, either parents or state agencies, who have custody of the child pending disposition. Once a new parent or parents have been recognized by the disposition decision, the appointment of counsel for the child should cease — unless specifically requested to continue by the new caretakers. They become the child's representative and thus become responsible for the child's legal care needs.

In divorce and separation proceedings, when parents are unable on their own to decide who shall have custody, justification for appointment of counsel has

---

[12]e.g., 11 Pa. Const. Stat. § 2223; 075.

[13]We now find insufficiently precise paragraph 30.4 of the Hampstead Haven Code: "Whenever an intervener seeks to alter a child's placement the child shall be made a party to the dispute. The child shall be represented by independent counsel." (Goldstein, Freud, and Solnit, *Beyond the Best Interests,* p. 100).

been established. In effect, invocation and adjudication collapse into a single transaction in which the parents, by failing to agree on a disposition, waive their claim to parental autonomy and thereby their claim to be the sole representatives of their child's interests. The child about whom his parents are in conflict thus requires independent representation to assure that his interests are treated as paramount in determining who shall have custody pending and upon final disposition. In families of more than one child, the continuity guideline would suggest that generally the same lawyer would represent all of the children, who share a community of interest in maintaining their ties with one another. Of course, there may be exceptional cases in which this presumption should be overcome. Again, once a final disposition is made each child should be presumed to have at least one autonomous parent who is responsible for sheltering them from direct contact with the law, for safeguarding their privacy and for generally representing their interests as a member of the family.

Once the court has imposed counsel for children, from whom is counsel to receive instructions? Court-imposed counsel may not look to the parents of the children. Those parents have voluntarily abdicated or have been temporarily or permanently disqualified as the exclusive representatives of their childrens' interests. Nor can counsel turn directly to the children who are represented, as counsel would to adult clients, for instructions. Children are by definition persons in need of adult caretakers who determine what is best for them. Nor may counsel draw upon personal child rearing preferences and seek to have them imposed upon the "client" without regard to the state's notion of what is best for children. It is to the court and to the legislature that counsel must turn for the guidance that would normally be received from autonomous parents who engage counsel to represent their children.

Like an autonomous parent, the court must advise counsel, as the child placement statutes might direct, for example, to determine what placement alternatives are most likely to maximize the opportunity for continuity of current or, if necessary, new relationships. And counsel might be required, for further example, with regard to both process and substance to press the court to take into account the child's sense of time, the limitation of experts to make long range predictions, and of courts to successfully monitor parent-child relationships. The court, like an autonomous parent, may find unconvincing and reject evidence or recommendations of counsel for the child.[14]

But, unlike the autonomous parent, the court may not have final say: counsel is empowered to appeal decisions believed to be in conflict with whatever standards the legislature may have established. However, the appointing court, like an autonomous parent, may dismiss counsel for failing to perform his or her duty, though unlike such parents, it cannot dismiss counsel without good cause. Finally, counsel appointed before adjudication for children in temporary emergency placement will be responsible for monitoring the child's care in order to assure that the court-ordered nurturing care is in fact being provided.

Thus, the court assumes, albeit temporarily, the authority of a parent to de-

---

[14]Child care agencies and disqualified parents continue to be parties to such proceedings. They of course can introduce whatever evidence the court determines is admissible and relevant and examine witnesses called by counsel for the child. (Smith v. Organization of Foster Families, 431 U.S. 816 [1977]).

termine the legal care needs of a child during that stage of the child placement process when the court must decide who is to be parent. The court, in a disposition proceeding, unlike the court in other civil proceedings, knows prior to the introduction of any evidence — prior to a hearing — which of the parties he will favor. The court, by statute, is obligated to favor the child and counsel for the child knows the client is supposed to win. That is another way of coming to understand why the court can generally be relied upon to serve as the parental substitute in relation to counsel. In order to compensate for the loss of full parental insulation, in order to protect the now-exposed child from judicial and child care agency policies and practices which might conflict with a particular child's interests, the court is obligated to appoint "independent" counsel to represent the child pending and until disposition.

Once disposition is final, once the court determines who is to be parent, the appointment of counsel for the child is terminated. Unless of course, legal services are requested by the "new" parent, his and the court's work are done. The court, in its selection of a custodial parent, is expressing the state's confidence that this particular adult has the capacity to fulfill the child's needs to be cared for, including the child's need to be protected from and represented before the law. To do otherwise as the Connecticut Superior Court did in *G. v. G.*[15] by imposing, as a condition of disposition, legal counsel for the child, is to undermine that confidence; it is to threaten rather than promote family integrity.

In *G. v. G.* Arthur, age 13, was represented by counsel appointed apparently at the request of the custodial parent who was seeking to prevent the noncustodial parent from resuming visitations which the court had recently suspended in the course of a battle which had been in and out of court for more than nine years. While the court denied the request for resumption of visits, it ordered the lawyer to continue to represent Arthur. The court observed:

> The attorney for the minor child has consented to remain as counsel of record. The child should feel free to consult with his attorney at any time pertaining to matters regarding his custody.

> Of course without further order of this court and with the consent of the plaintiff-mother (the custodial parent) *and* the consent of the minor child through his attorney, visitation may be resumed under appropriate arrangement. . . .

> It should be made clear that consent of both the plaintiff-mother and the minor child or an order of this court must be obtained before there can be a resumption of visitation.

In interposing an attorney between Arthur and his mother, the custodial parent, the court undermines their opportunity to relate directly to one another. It is the attorney's consent, not the mother's, which the court has obtained for the appointment. Arthur is thus deprived of a parent upon whom he can rely to respond to his wishes, to determine his needs, and to represent his interests — even to decide whether he requires legal assistance. His mother cannot, for

---

[15]G. v. G., Conn. Super. Ct. No. 11 28 46 (April 6, 1977) (unreported opinion).

example, make him visit his father or grant him permission to do so. She would first have to obtain the concurrence of "Arthur's counsel" or permission from the court to overcome counsel's objection. And were counsel to decide, over her objection, that visits should be resumed counsel may seek judicial supervention of her judgment. By imposing conditions of this kind, the court places itself and counsel between parent and child; it subverts rather than safeguards the child's critical need for an autonomous parent. The occasions for court orders as intrusive and as divisive as that in *G. v. G.* would, of course, be minimized, if not eliminated, in a child placement system which observed the least detrimental alternative standard and made all placements permanent, unconditional and final, except for emergency, institutional and truly temporary foster care. Under the current system the only continuity the Arthurs can anticipate is the continuity of state intrusion.

Emancipating Children for Legal Service Purposes

In bringing this inquiry to a close, I want to shift its focus for a moment from who among competing adults may represent a child's interests before the law to circumstances when children should be treated as adults in their own right, with the authority to engage and to instruct counsel to pursue what they — the emancipated "children" — believe to be in their own best interests. Of course counsel for children, whether engaged by autonomous parents or by judge, as substitute parent, may be advised to take into account the children's wishes in representing their interests. But such children, because they are children — not adults — are without authority to engage or dismiss their counsel. The question is whether and when children should be given such authority free of adult control. As "adults" such children would be presumed both competent and free to determine their own placement needs and to arrange to meet them. Put another way the question becomes, under what circumstances should the law presume that a child is as competent as an adult to be free of the care and control of parents.

Any answer to this question which would qualify a minor as an adult must provide a standard of emancipation which is as impersonal and as nonjudgmental as is chronological age for establishing adult, nonchild, status. For the emancipation to be real, all children in the category, for example, children institutionalized at their parents' request or children who are pregnant, would have to be deemed qualified to refuse as well as to accept the service and advice of counsel. It would be fiction were an emancipation statute to cover only children who "choose" to accept counsel or who on a case-by-case basis are found to be, for example, "mature enough" to decide. That would only transfer from the parent to the judge, not to the child, the prerogative and responsibility to determine when to consult and whether to abide by the child's wishes. It would not be too difficult to draft a real emancipation statute which would meet the fair warning and power restraint requirements of such a ground for terminating parent-child relationships. But I will not make the effort because I do not believe that there are any circumstances which justify emancipating children to meet their own legal care needs. Just because they are children, just because they need to be represented by parents, just because the purpose of the child placement process is to secure or restore for every child an uninterrupted opportunity to be represented by parents they cannot, by definition, be free of parental (or, if parents have been disqualified, free of judicial) review and control in determining their need for legal assistance.

In *In re Gault*[16] the United States Supreme Court extended the right to counsel to children charged with delinquency; but it did not emancipate them for legal-services purposes. This decision is often misread not to mean emancipation but to mean that parents of such children are not to "be relied upon to protect the infant's interests." That erroneous reading has been used to disqualify, without process, parents as the representatives of their child and to deprive children, without process, of their parents' representation.

Gault means and should be read to mean that a child in a juvenile delinquency proceeding will not be deprived of the right to legal representation because it is a civil, not a criminal proceeding, or solely because his parents are financially unable to afford counsel. Indeed, the parents of young Gault initiated the action in order to assure that they not be denied the right, as his representatives — as insulating adults — to provide their child with the legal representation they believed he needed and was entitled to by a right which they were unwilling to waive.[17] The *Gault* court held that: "The child and his parents must be notified of the child's right to be represented by counsel retained by them, or if they are unable to afford counsel, that counsel will be appointed to represent the child."

Looked at more broadly, and to return to the primary focus of this inquiry, *Gault* was an attempt to reduce, to mitigate, the extent to which the state, through one part of its child placement system, had come to undermine the family and the role of parents in relation to their children. The decision grew out of the Court's recognition that the juvenile justice system, though initially intended to meet the special and individual needs of children caught up in an otherwise heartless, nonrehabilitative system of criminal law, had, by the time young Gault entered it, become in many ways as punitive and as "inhumane" as its adult counterpart. But it was worse, because the child was deprived of the insulation from direct contact with law that parents hope to provide. Thus rather than extend the "good intentions" of juvenile court judges by letting them — or other state representatives — play parent to the child, *Gault* would have let the child's own parents make the decisions about what he needs. There is no hint in *Gault,* and it would run contrary to its tenor, that an attorney could independently represent the child over the parents' objection and prior to their disqualification as the exclusive representatives of his interests. Protection of the family, protection of the child from the state — not from his parents — is central to the holding in *Gault* and indeed to what I propose be the

---

[16]*In re* Gault, 387 U.S. 1, 35, 41 (1967).
[17]Application of Gault, 90 Ariz. 181, 407 P. 2d 670 (en banc 1965).

criteria for the appointment and function of counsel for children. If that notion takes firm root, not only in the jurisprudence but also in the custom and practice of child placement law, the psychological well-being of children will be served.

Acknowledgement

This article draws on material prepared for a book which I am writing with Anna Freud and Albert J. Solnit entitled *Before the Best Interests of the Child*. In addition to my collaborators, I am indebted to Sonja Goldstein and to my students at Yale Law School who participated in the Family Law Seminar, particularly David De Wolf, Paula Herman, Carol Larson, Martha Minow, and Donn P. Pickett for their assistance.

Comments on Goldstein's "Psychoanalysis and a Jurisprudence of Child Placement"

Commentator: Quentin Rae-Grant*

Professor Goldstein has had many years of obviously enjoyable and fruitful collaboration with two eminent psychoanalysts. The distillate of their experience over many years I presumed, as did many others, to have culminated in the book *Beyond the Best Interests of the Child*.[1] This relatively brief, conceptually sound, and in most cases practical approach to one of the most thorny issues has certainly been one, if not the most, influential publication over these many last years. Few, if any, who work with children, parents or families are not both aware of, and increasingly guided by, the precepts contained in that volume. Perhaps its greatest contribution has been to move aside a myth that had bedevilled both psychiatry and the law, namely, the frantic search for "the best interests of the child." It acknowledged what had been operating for a long time but could not be openly stated, namely, that in many situations there was no best answer. It made it possible to seek, without guilt for failing to meet that unobtainable objective, the arrangement which was least detrimental. As well, it brought the interests of the child into focus, namely, that they required attention and hearing, a differential value depending on age and maturity but requiring consideration alongside the wishes of the adults. Finally, it was clearly enunciated that in certain impossible situations an arbitrary decision (but at least a decision) with regard to custody and access was perhaps the crucial issue and that of most importance for the child. It is therefore most heartening and most tantalizing to know that the three same collaborators are in the process of preparing a further examination of these issues to be entitled *Before the Best Interests of the Child*. To both of these tasks Professor Goldstein brings a point of view which encompasses experience in the law and experience in clinical practice. This double qualification is rare and probably the envy of many. However, perhaps it also brings something of a danger, that any presentation will be viewed by the clinician as too legally oriented, and by the lawyer as too influenced by clinical considerations. We shall see.

Professor Goldstein's emphasis on the clear separation of the process of invocation, process of adjudication and the process of disposition goes far towards clearing up the confusion that frequently arises when the three are intermingled. Professor Goldstein is also to be commended, particularly when he speaks as a lawyer, for avoiding the all too easy assumption that inattention or

*Professor and Vice-Chairman, Department of Psychiatry, University of Toronto; and Psychiatrist-in-Chief, Hospital for Sick Children, Toronto, Canada.
[1] J. Goldstein, A Freud, and A. J. Solnit, *Beyond the Best Interests of the Child*. (New York: Free Press, 1973).

unfairness to children can always be remedied by appointment of a child advocate or child's own counsel. Perhaps one consequence of such an appointment is to improve the quality of the paperwork and the care put into its preparation. What remains to be demonstrated is that it improves the eventual outcome as far as the child's life is concerned. Indeed at times it may be simply a substituting of one set of values for another — the values depending on discipline, orientation and personal persuasion of those who act in this capacity. Neither representatives of the more legal nor the more clinical side of these issues have any particular demonstrated right to claim predictive accuracy with regard to the crucial issue of the parenting capacities of the various alternatives. All who are engaged in this capacity recognize that the ability to predict who will best carry these out, and in what way, is at the best an informed guess. By defining when, why, for what purposes and for how long the child's counsel may function, Professor Goldstein is attempting not only to safeguard the child but also the integrity of the nurturing unit. Particularly important is the recognition that sometimes solutions proposed solve one problem while creating simultaneously another set, and that simple prescriptions are inappropriate for complex issues. In his paper he tries to steer the fine line between the need for state intervention and clinical do-goodiness.

It would be obviously inappropriate for me to comment on this from a legal point of view. I shall confine myself in the discussion to some questions raised within me as a clinician. I do this particularly because the phrase "the best interest of the child" has in so many instances been used as a justification for doing things which in the end may turn out bo be anything but the best interests of the child. Thus, the less formal and more rehabilitative approaches of juvenile delinquency acts were meant to improve the lot of children, but simultaneously deprived them of a number of rights to which they had been entitled.

The Gault ruling, to which Professor Goldstein refers, was arrived at by way of a Writ of Habeas Corpus, two years of litigation, and the Supreme Court ruling before the boy was released in 1967.[2] His offence was a number of obscene calls (or what at that time were regarded as obscene calls), the content and tenor of which, however, can be seen today in many easily available and obviously popular magazines of a particular genre. The decision restored to the child certain rights, e.g., to cross-examine and confront hostile witnesses, the right to avoid self-incrimination, which had become lost in the process of trying to care in a more considerate way for those of younger years. However, and it is this point to which Professor Goldstein takes considerable exception, it introduces as a right the availability to the child on a rather broad basis of his own legal counsel.

In Canada, an Amendment to the Criminal Code passed in 1892 asserted that children should have a different trial from adults, one that stresses rehabilitation and privacy.[3] The juvenile process was to espouse a more liberal choice of disposition and the emphasis was shifted towards a therapeutic mode. In return for this privilege however, ironically, the child was stripped of most of the liberalities of the adult court. He was not accorded the right to bail, counsel, or

---

[2] *In Re Gault,* 387 U.S. 1, 35, 41 (1967).
[3] *The Juvenile Delinquents Act,* R.S.C. 1970, c.J-3.

the right to confront his accusers. A review opinion sixty years later reads as follows:

> The original Juvenile Court Act as enacted . . . was devised to afford the juvenile protections *in addition* to those he already possessed. . . . Before this legislative enactment, the juvenile was subject to the same punishment for an offence as an adult. It follows logically that in the absence of such legislation, the juvenile would be entitled to the same constitutional guarantees and safeguards as an adult. If this be true, then the only possible reason for the Juvenile Court Act was to affort the juvenile safeguards in addition to those he already possessed. The Legislature's intent was to enlarge, not to diminish, these protections.[4]

While obviously, then, I have the highest admiration for Professor Goldstein's paper and find little to quarrel with it as a legal document, there are a few concerns which I would like to raise. Deliberately and understandably there is no attempt to define a family, yet today I would suggest that this word is rapidly losing much of its original meaning and acquiring many new ones. In approaching the rights of parents, biological or otherwise, or parent substitutes, are we then in danger of using an evolutionary approach to the mounting problems of a revolutionary change in our society? This question is particularly timely in Canada and in this Province where major changes in both federal and provincial legislation are in the process of discussion and development* and where the concept of a unified family court is being tried in a selected number of areas. In light of our present knowledge of an increasingly early age of physical and social maturity, can we continue to talk of children and adolescents as if the arbitrary chronological dividing line, be it 16 or 18 according to jurisdiction and different acts, has any real meaning in terms of the people involved? Rather, it would seem that this might be a matter of management simplicity. This acceptance of the chronological definition of the status of the child troubles me as we have gone through an era when emancipated youth and those who spoke on their behalf fought hard to have privileges recognized, but never had them accepted as rights and are now in real danger of a gradual attrition of what was in practice gained, but which was never accepted within official codes.

Professor Goldstein's set of premises recommending the least intervention, the least intrusive intervention for the least possible time is certainly concordant with some principles for community mental health practice that Hollister and myself tried to outline under the title of "Principles of Parsimony."[5] These principles can be briefly defined as follows:
1. The least disruptive intervention is the first treatment of choice.
2. The least separation from family and job will be sought.
3. The least expensive treatment will be used first.

---

*The *Family Law Reform Act* of Ontario became effective on March 31, 1978. (ed.)

[4]Nicholas N. Kittrie, *Right to be Different: Deviance and Enforced Therapy.* (Baltimore: Johns Hopkins, 1972).

[5]W. G. Hollister and Q. Rae-Grant, "The Principles of Parsimony in Mental Health Center Operations," *Canada's Mental Health.* 20(1) (1972):18–24.

4. The least extensive intervention will be used first.

5. The least trained intervenors will be used first.

But overriding all of these is the consideration of effectiveness. The analogous concern in the legal intervention with children would certainly seem to be the factor of time. Particularly for younger children, at least as important as knowing what decision is made is having that decision finalized and therefore having a clarification of that to which they must now adjust. The longer this era of uncertainty lasts, would not the psychoanalyst agree, the more potential are the deleterious effects.

One particular sentence in Goldstein's case vignette did trouble me greatly — "Charlie mistakenly sought to allocate to himself the status of adult." While this may be appropriate and understandable for a ten year-old, is it equally so for a fourteen or fifteen year-old, and what other than practice would determine (or should determine) that this is a mistaken action? The principle that parents know best is unfortunately sadly torn to shreds by the furiously fought battles in custody and access cases. The problems arise not only in cases where there is dispute, but also in cases where a very careful and complex arrangement has been arrived at by mutual agreement or by the pressure of one partner and the surrender of the other. This is supplied to the court for ratification but too often provides continuing opportunities, indeed invitations, for the two parents to go "at it," for the children to be go-betweens, and for everyone to grind each other into small and rather miserable pieces.

Finally, I was struck by the absence of the use and reliance on what I would call outcome information. In fact, perhaps it is not by accident that a commonality exists between law and psychoanalysis, as the development of both fields use a closely similar process. The law (if my crude information is correct) develops by precedent and the reverent quotation thereof. In psychoanalysis and much of clinical psychiatry, the equivalent process is deference to the opinions of those who have written before, or one's personal experience with cases; two sources which are necessary but not perhaps sufficient for the most enlightened of changes. Again, speaking as a clinician, I am concerned at the appalling dearth of information as to what happens with regard to children who are handled in different ways and by different judgements. Surely by now, with rising divorce and separation rates, we should have accumulated hard facts which would tell us which children are in danger, at which age, which things work, which things do not work. Yet, to the best of my knowledge, we have to be content with studies such as that of Wallerstein and Kelly which deal with case numbers in the middle thirties,[6] when our divorce rate in some jurisdictions is now over 50% of the rate of marriages. While I would be the first to admit that clinical practice is resistant to change of a research nature by about a factor of 5 to 10 years, would it be unfair to say that perhaps this is a little bit faster than the use of similar information to effect change in legal procedure and legislation? Where information can be collected, surely it is our obligation and duty to look at the consequences of our actions and not merely to debate their niceties.

---

[6] J. S. Wallerstein and J. B. Kelly, "The Effects of Parental Divorce: Experiences of the Preschool Child," *Journal of the American Academy of Child Psychiatry* 14 (1975):600–616.

Both psychiatry and the law are, I think, at the moment crying out for information of this type, information that would fill in the gaps in our knowledge, e.g., the impact of divorce, various arrangements of custody and access, the changes in these over the years and with increasing age of children and what really happens. How often, in fact, do the carefully worked out arrangements simply dissipate with rather rapid changes and passage of time? This is in no way to denigrate what we can learn from the past or from the wisdom of those who have gone before. It is a plea to combine that with empirical evidence which may confirm but may also refute our assumptions.

Comments on Goldstein's "Psychoanalysis and a Jurisprudence of Child Placement"

Commentator: Bernard Dickens*

Professor Goldstein's paper presents a disquieting challenge, since it explores the point at which society's well-meaning urge to protect children may threaten the substance or at least the quality of family life, which society has no less strong an urge to protect. It questions the means by which we determine the welfare of children, and compels us to face the possibility that liberal instincts to furnish protection may be totalitarian, and that identification of dysfunctional families may not be sufficiently tolerant or accommodating of parents who simply dissent.

The challenge is timely in the evolution of Canadian thinking on the legal representation of children, since pending federal legislation on young offenders proposes a more rigid legal form of trial of juvenile suspects,[1] of which legal representation is a significant element.[2] Family Advocates were introduced in British Columbia in 1974, with duties and discretions on child representation,[3] the government of Alberta is considering proposals for systematic representation of juveniles,[4] and in Ontario the Attorney General's Committee on the Representation of Children is actively considering pilot projects to implement its widely approved recommendation of June 1977[5] that both delinquency defendants and children claimed to be in need of protection, as defined in Part II of the Child Welfare Act,[6] be afforded legal representation. The committee's terms of reference were widened earlier this year to include children liable to be immediately affected by the outcome of custody and access hearings. The concept of the right to legal representation of children has spread so recently in Canada, that non-representation is still coming to be regarded as a misfortune and fault in the system of legal process, rather than as an independent legal right of parents, and of children themselves.

The thesis of optimal legal services for children in litigation affecting their future is fundamentally challenged by Professor Goldstein's antithesis of mini-

---

*Faculty of Law, University of Toronto, Canada.

[1] See Solicitor General of Canada, "Highlights of the Proposed New Legislation for Young Offenders," *Criminal Reports (New Series)* 37 (1977): 113–146.

[2] "The proposals provide that a young person must be represented at his trial by a lawyer, unless the judge of the youth court is satisfied that no lawyer is reasonably available. In such instances, the judge would allow a young person to be assisted by a responsible adult." Ibid., p. 119.

[3] Unified Family Court Act, S.B.C. 1974, c. 99, s.8.

[4] See generally Bernard M. Dickens, "Representing the Child in the Courts" in I. F. G. Baxter and M. Eberts, eds., *The Child and the Courts* (Toronto: Carswell Co., 1978), pp. 273–298.

[5] *Report of the Committee on the Representation of Children in the Provincial Court (Family Division)* (Toronto: Ministry of the Attorney General, 1977).

[6] R.S.O. 1970, c.64, Part II Protection and Care of Neglected Children; see s.20(1)(b).

mal state intervention in families, and the dilemma of synthesis is rendered more acute by recognizing that both thesis and antithesis represent in themselves goals worthy of communal respect and advancement. The search for means of accommodation between these incompatible virtues compels us to face the implications of the underlying propositions. Professor Goldstein has stated the postulates that:

> To be a *child* is to be at risk, dependent, and without capacity or authority to decide what is 'best' for oneself.
> To be an *adult* is to be a risktaker, independent, and with capacity and authority to decide and to do what is 'best' for oneself.
> To be an *adult who is a parent* is to be presumed in law to have the capacity, authority, and responsibility to determine and to do what is good for one's children.[7]

If an adult is "a risktaker," a parent is an adult who may take a risk for a child. The risk is the risk of suffering or causing harm, and the right to decide on risk includes the right to be wrong. Society must bear the anguish of letting parents be mistaken, in order to allow them the autonomous capacity to exercise correct judgment. Family integrity may exist at a price its children may be called upon to pay.

Professor Goldstein asks at what point what passes for the wisdom of the community may impose itself over individual parental decision-taking on behalf of children, and thereby may undermine or diminish the role of parents. His answer lies in the realm not so much of substance, as of process;[8] that is, not in defining the limits of parental authority as such, but in requiring due legal process of proof of indications that a given family unit is dysfunctional. Only when the family is disqualified by due process of law or by extreme emergency from the exercise of autonomy may parental choice be superseded.

The ordering of priorities proposed in Professor Goldstein's paper is that, first, parents exercise choice as to legal representation of their children involved in or affected by litigation, and at this point the right to select representation, however supplied, ranks no more than equally with the right to select not to have representation, from whatever source it might be available. Secondly, if legal process discloses parental guardianship of children to have been inadequate, by reference to factors other than denial of legal representation, the issue of the future best interests of the children arises for determination by the court, and for this purpose the children may be given legal representation, even over parental objection.

This proposed sequence of decision-taking regarding legal representation is fully compatible with decision-taking regarding other interests of children, such as health care and education. A parent initially determines a child's health

---

[7] Joseph Goldstein, "Medical Care for the Child at Risk: On State Supervention of Parental Autonomy," *Yale Law Journal* 86 (1977): 645. (Italics in original).

[8] The observation in his paper regarding legal representation is consistent with his view regarding medical care, that "the law then must limit the state to determining by some relatively objective standard *who* is entitled to decide, not *what* specific decision is to be preferred in a particular case nor whether a specific child has the 'wisdom' to make a choice." Ibid., p. 663.

needs, but under the provincial Child Welfare Act a child may be found in need of protection by a court:

> Where the person in whose charge he is neglects or refuses to provide or obtain proper medical, surgical or other recognized remedial care or treatment necessary for his health or well-being, or refuses to permit such care or treatment to be supplied to the child when it is recommended by a legally qualified medical practitioner.[9]

Medical opinions on health care or treatment may differ, but this formula requires observance of a more objective standard of care than an individual parent may apply. The law thereby gives advance notice, or fair warning, of what its standards are. This cannot guarantee the child's welfare, of course, and may indeed submit a particular child to the risks of drug administrations, innoculations or surgery a parent resists. Its potential for oppressive use is clear,[10] especially against adherents to beliefs the general community considers eccentric, but we trust that improper use of the formula will be only an aberration, and that it will set a general minimum standard of health care beneath which parental practice, whether by neglect or choice, will not sink without correction.

Similarly, in a recent English case,[11] a dedicated parent opposed to the state system of education and unable to afford to send his child to a fee-paying separate school, sent him to none. The child was held to be in need of care, although the parent's degree of concern for the child was perhaps praiseworthy. On an objective scale, the parent was found to be mistaken, and this justified judicial intervention between parent and child to give the child an institutional means of education.[12]

Again, extension of this precedent may generate fears of abuse, since it may provide means to regulate parental instruction of their children in social and political philosophies, and, for instance, in theistic and atheistic convictions.[13] We may perhaps be compelled to ask not whether due process of law has been observed in these cases, but whether due process of law is enough. The oppression of intolerant law is not relieved in being applied by due process. Professor Goldstein's vision clearly embraces this perception, but let me return to his immediate text.

Before expressing certain reservations about application of the proposed ordering of priorities where legal representation is concerned, I want to applaud the great virtue of Professor Goldstein's paper in emphasizing the necessary distinction in litigation affecting children and juveniles between adjudication and disposition. There is evidence, particularly but not only in the proportion of guilty pleas to delinquency charges and of parental concurrence in protec-

---

[9] Note 6 above, s. 20(1)(b)(x).

[10] See John J. Paris, "Compulsory Medical Treatment and Religious Freedom: Whose Law Shall Prevail?" *University of San Francisco Law Review* 10 (1975): 1–35.

[11] *In re S. (A Minor) (Care Order: Education)*, [1977] 3 W.L.R. 575 (C.A.).

[12] Ontario's Child Welfare Act, note 6 above, renders "a child who, without sufficient cause, habitually absents himself from his home or school" in need of protection; see s.20(1)(b)(ix).

[13] See Judith Areen, "Intervention Between Parent and Child: A Reappraisal of the State's Role in Child Neglect and Abuse Cases," *Georgetown Law Journal* 63 (1975): 887–937, and Michael S. Wald, "State Intervention on Behalf of 'Neglected' Children: A Search for Realistic Standards," *Stanford Law Review* 27 (1975): 985–1040.

tion proceedings, that the adjudication stage of litigation may be discounted or compressed in judicial enthusiasm to do the good for a child which a court considers it can achieve at disposition.[14] A court conscious of its means to give a child a better material and/or emotional environment than he has may be impatient of obstacles to implementing its remedial programme. If the precondition of implementation is a formal finding of delinquency or of a need for protection, the court may become motivated to reach such a finding. This is accentuated in that delinquency and protection proceedings seem so often to involve the most needful children in the community;[15] children of low-income homes, single-parent or disordered families, disadvantaged groups, and children of homes which have experienced many revolutions in the cycle of welfare dependency. The right on adjudication to acquittal, and to remain unprotected by the courts, may be considered cheap when valued against the rich promise of the better life to which disposition may appear to lead.

Yet in noting how matters relevant in court to adjudication may interact with issues of disposition, we may feel a little discomfort at having a child's interest in legal representation protected only after adverse adjudication has been reached. To elaborate on this source of my personal reservations about Professor Goldstein's proposal, I want to distinguish between delinquency hearings, protection hearings and hearings concerning the custody of and access to children upon termination of marital unity. My reservations are more pragmatic than doctrinal, since I accept the initial premises from which Professor Goldstein advances his reasoning. I feel and fear, however, that the practical exceptions to his doctrine may so overwhelm the areas of its applicability that for operational purposes his policy preference will only infrequently appear to prevail.

Delinquency proceedings in Canada, unlike certain of such proceedings in the United States, are clearly criminal in character,[16] despite the welfare rhetoric in which many of their procedures are conducted. They fall within the criminal law power of the federal government,[17] and the young person accused is a criminal defendant, facing the charge of having committed a delinquency which, under pending legislation, will be confined to an offence against federal law or subordinate legislation made under federal provisions.[18] The parents are not parties, and the quality of their parenting is not immediately relevant to whether or not the offence was committed. Indications of the calibre of the young person's home life almost unavoidably seep into the adjudication process, however, perhaps with the prejudicial effect of showing him to conform to the profile or stereotype of the "young offender."

---

[14] See Jeffrey S. Leon, "The Development of Canadian Juvenile Justice: A Background for Reform" *Osgoode Hall Law Journal* 15 (1977): 71–106, and Katherine Catton and Jeffrey S. Leon, "Legal Representation and the Proposed Young Persons in Conflict With the Law Act." Ibid., pp. 107–135.

[15] See Judith Areen and Michael S. Wald, note 13 above.

[16] Legal difficulties attributable to the noncriminal, *parens patriae* concept of juvenile court jurisdiction in the United States were identified by Monrad G. Paulsen in "The Expanding Horizons of Legal Services," *West Virginia Law Review* 67 (1965): 267–290.

[17] The Juvenile Delinquents Act, R.S.C. 1970, c.J-3, was enacted under s.91(27) of the British North America Act, 1867, 30 & 31 Vict., c.3. See generally Larry Wilson, "Juvenile Justice and the Criminal Law Power," *Saskatchewan Law Review* 41 (1977): 253–267.

[18] See note 1 above, p. 116.

To require demonstration of parental shortcoming as a pre-condition of appointing counsel to aid the young defendant over parental opposition may be to go too far in pursuit of a non-interventionist philosophy. Legal representation differs from health care and, for instance, education, in that parental choice is exercised regarding these services before the suspicion can arise that the standard of parental performance falls short of the objective minimum standard society requires to be observed. Further, the harm of inadequate supply of services is usually reversible upon identification and proof by due process of law (although cases of irreversible health damage are pitiful and tragic). When a young person unrepresented at his parent's wish is adjudicated a criminal offender, however, there is no way to annul the judgement on that ground or to have the case re-tried;[19] his very means of appeal may be excluded by the absence of counsel. It is ironically the case that legal recourse is greater against the ineffective or incompetent assistance of counsel than against the absence of counsel by choice.[20] The state, in the form of the Crown prosecutor, rarely denies itself the benefit of legal counsel, and it seems unreasonable for a parent with the opportunity to obtain counsel for his child, whether by payment or otherwise, to elect to allow the child to go unrepresented.

Accordingly, I would propose that Professor Goldstein's principle of family integrity be balanced against the prospect of counsel for the child being appointed against parental opposition, by affording the parent the opportunity to satisfy the court, in a preliminary proceeding, perhaps when the date for trial is being fixed, or at the commencement of the proceedings and before the defendant's plea is taken, that his preference for non-representation of the young defendant should prevail. If he can show that his responsibility as a parent is being appropriately discharged, his choice in his relationship with his child may be preserved. The importance of the child's interest in being represented, I would submit, justifies reversing the normal onus and requiring the parent to establish the merit of his preference, and to show that he is not acting arbitrarily, negligently or maliciously. It may follow that when he has himself instigated or expressly favoured the delinquency proceedings, his preference may be superseded without further process.

The same may be applicable in protection proceedings, brought by a children's aid society to show the child to be in need of protection, when the parent complies in the proceedings[21] or fails to appear as respondent. Protection proceedings are against parents, the children not being parties to the litigation. It may seem that parents not themselves contesting the application for a court order will not sponsor legal representation of their child, and will find no purpose served in allowing representation even at no cost to themselves. It should not follow upon their declining or failing to show cause for non-representation

---

[19] The prevailing underlying attitude appears to be that, "The fundamental justice for an accused is a fair trial; counsel is not always a necessary concomitant to a fair trial," per Clements, J. A. in *Re Gilberg and The Queen,* 53 D.L.R. (3rd) 441 (Alta. S.C., App. D.) at p. 453.

[20] See Asher D. Grunis, "Incompetence of Defence Counsel in Criminal Cases," *The Criminal Law Quarterly* 16 (1974): 288–306.

[21] Ontario's Child Welfare Act, see note 6 above, automatically renders a child in need of protection "who is brought, with the consent of the person in whose charge he is, before a judge to be dealt with under this Part" (i.e. Part II of the Act); see s.20(1)(b)(i). Accordingly, adjudication is pre-determined by the mode of initiation of the proceedings.

that a lawyer will then be appointed. It may mean, however, that a judge, duty counsel, agent of the Official Guardian, public defender or other lawyer appointed to the task should screen the case to determine if representation is desirable, and make arrangements if it appears to be.[22]

When a parent contests the application for a finding of need for protection, Professor Goldstein's proposal may prevail, permitting the parent to decide upon supplying or seeking separate representation for the child in the proceedings up to adjudication. At present, Ontario's Child Welfare Act does not expressly permit representation of the child, of course, but a Bill shortly to go before the Legislature is intended to change this position.[23] If at adjudication the court finds the child not to be an abused child, the matter ends there, but if, on the other hand, the child's need for protection is established, the court will then go on to consider the appropriate disposition, and whether the child should be legally represented during the disposition proceedings. Since parental deficiency has at that point been found by due process, it would appear that Professor Goldstein's condition has been satisfied for a court-ordered representative to be appointed for the child, at the determination of the court's own screening mechanism.

Delinquency and protection proceedings may be instigated by or concurred in by parents, but most often they are brought by agencies outside the family. Custody and access proceedings are different, however, in that they originate within the family, at the point of its fragmentation. The stable, caring, nurturing domestic unit that Professor Goldstein has argued should be trusted to protect its children from legal contact, may in this case be about to be dismembered by legal process initiated by the parents, and determination of the children's destiny unavoidably falls to the courts.

Professor Goldstein has proposed that separate legal representation of the child should not be considered until it is shown that the child's future relationship with his parents may have to be modified. Pursuit of separation or divorce proceedings may show this axiomatically, unless they are designed simply to allow the court formally to suspend or to bury a legal marriage already dead as a social fact. The issue in custody hearings may not be whether either parent is fit or unfit to have custody of or access to the child, but what the future relationship of each parent to the child is to be. Each parent will have a preference, but this is not necessarily compatible with the child's best interests.[24] Neither parent may seem likely to be willing to provide a lawyer for the child to resist that preference, however, or to allow a lawyer to be supplied to the child from elsewhere. The parent may appear to have a conflicting interest with the child, even when the parent wishes for custody of the child and the child wants to be

---

22 See note 5 above, para. 49, pp. 30–32.

23 To amend s. 20(2) of the current Child Welfare Act, see note 6 above, to provide, "Where a child is not represented by counsel or agent in an application under this Part or at any stage of the proceedings, a judge, if he is of the opinion that such representation is desirable, may appoint counsel to represent the child in the proceedings or allow the child to be represented in the proceedings by such other responsible person whom the judge deems suitable."

24 See Doris J. Freed and Henry H. Foster, "The Shuffled Child and Divorce Court," *Trial* 10 (May/ June 1974): 26. The authors note that, under developing no-fault divorce concepts, there is "an enhanced tendency to treat custodial . . . problems in a *pro forma* fashion" (p. 41).

placed with that parent. Independent assessment of the child's need for legal representation may therefore be appropriate, although the role of a lawyer appointed in that situation raises important issues time does not allow to be considered at present.[25]

The need for separate representation of the child may be no less great when the parents have agreed between themselves as to custody of and access to the child. If the proceedings are designed simply to regularize in law the social fact of earlier marriage breakdown, when the child's existing domestic environment and relationships will continue unchanged, legal representation may, of course, be unnecessary. When the parents have agreed about a new environment for the child, however, it does not follow that this agreement serves the child's best interests, but the parents will be unlikely to consider supplying an independent lawyer for the child to monitor the terms of their agreement, perhaps arranged by their own legal representatives. The agreement may reflect hard bargaining between the parents, with, for instance, a father giving up a custody claim and access rights in return for relief from obligations of financial support, or a mother releasing a claim over one child in order to retain undisturbed custody and support of another. These agreements, which at the same time may appear both mercenary and heart-rending, are liable to judicial scrutiny, but this does not necessarily promote their inspection through the eyes of the child. A lawyer for the child, meaning a lawyer *for* the child and not merely *to* the child, may be necessary in a way the parents cannot see, and have an incentive to resist; and all of Professor Goldstein's preconditions for the imposition of counsel over parental opposition may be satisfied.

I trust that, in conclusion, I may be allowed to go one step beyond Professor Goldstein's paper and mention one further relevant area where independent legal representation of a child may be desirable over parental refusal to provide or allow such representation. Where parents instigate the committal of their child to a mental health facility, the child's means of legal challenge to that committal, and to continued detention, are clearly compromised.[26] Here again, Professor Goldstein's conditions for the appointment of counsel may appear to be satisfied; the child's circumstances are clearly being changed, and the parents have yielded their role of protecting the child from involvement with the state and with the legal system. From the child's perspective, moreover, the circumstances may have taken on the character of an emergency in that he has been committed to an institution on the initiative of his only source of protection against such committal. A case may be made for requiring facilities admitting

---

[25] Much discussion of legal representation of children in Canada begs the fundamental issue of what function the lawyer is to serve. It must be decided, for instance, whether he is to represent the wishes of the child, or the interests of the child. See generally Bernard M. Dickens, "Legal Responses to Child Abuse in Canada," *Canadian Journal of Family Law* 1 (1978): pp. 87–125, and note 4 above. See also Robert H. Mnookin "American Custody Law: A Framework for Analysis" in the very useful *Proceedings of the University of Wisconsin Conference on Child Advocacy,* ed. Jack C. Westman (Madison: U. of Wisconsin – Extension Health Sciences Unit, 1976), pp. 123–150.

[26] See " 'Voluntary' Admission of Children to Mental Hospitals: A Conflict of Interest between Parent and Child," *Maryland Law Review* 36 (1976):153–181, and Jan. N. Holladay, "Due Process Limitations on Parental Rights to Commit Children to Mental Institutions," *University of Colorado Law Review* 48 (1977): 235–266.

children at the instigation of their parents to serve immediate notice upon the Official Guardian. Comparable issues may arise when parents have not taken an initiative, but have just passively concurred in committal, but these lie beyond our present concerns.

Major Issues in the Polish Mental Health Legislation Draft Proposal

Stanislaw Dabrowski*

Mental Health care in Poland is provided in accordance with directives issued by the Minister of Health and Social Welfare and is therefore not governed by a legal Mental Health Code. Numerous attempts to enact a Mental Health Act in Poland have met with insurmountable difficulties. The first such attempt occurred over a half a century ago and occasioned as much controversy and heated debate as subsequent proposals to promulgate a Mental Health Act. The last proposal, prior to the one currently under consideration, was defeated in 1970 in the final stages of the legislative process.

Our prior experience, and in particular the lessons learned from the ill-fated Bill of 1970, convinced us that the ultimate enactment of a Mental Health Act would require extensive public discussions beforehand, within and between interested groups such as psychiatrists, lawyers, psychologists, sociologists, patients and their families, and the general public. Open debate focusing upon controversial issues was considered the most expedient method to crystalize the primary assumptions underlying the new legislation, for overcoming resistance, and for developing a common alliance between competing parties.

The draft of the proposed Act, which I have the honor to present, is a totally new legislative proposal.[1] It attempts to overcome objections raised against the preceding proposal as well as to incorporate the suggestions and recommendations which surfaced during the year-long discussion on "the Main Theses of the Proposed Mental Health Act" which were published in June 1974.[2]

Public Debate Concerning the Draft Proposal

The discussions which followed publication of "The Theses" occurred primarily in the mass media and in psychiatric circles. It is noteworthy that the judiciary and the Office of the District Attorney were represented at all meetings sponsored by the Polish Psychiatric Association for reviewing the Draft. On a smaller scale, the Proposal was discussed during meetings of various professional, legal, sociological and religious associations.

Commentaries in the mass media, broad in scope and fervent in content, were avidly followed by the Polish public. Hundreds of letters were received by editors of weekly and monthly magazines, the Radio and Television Commit-

---

*Director, Psychoneurological Institute of Warsaw, Poland.

[1] Projekt ustawy o ochronie zdrowia psychicznego. Piata weraja redakcyjna. Instytut Psychoneurologiczny, Warszawa 1977.

[2] Tezy dotyczace prawnej regulacji ochrony zdrowia psychicznego Min. Zdr. i Op. Spol., Warszawa 1974.

tee, and members of the Commission of Experts which formulated the Draft Proposal. Daily newspapers joined with socio-literary and legal journals to debate the issues. While radio and television coverage tended to be popularized and informational in its thrust, discussions in the press examined the merits of the proposed regulations more deeply.

Several conclusions could be drawn from the articles in the press, which numbered well over one hundred. The need for a Polish Mental Health Act was strongly supported. It was generally agreed that "The Theses" differed from previous proposals in that they were presented for public discussion and thus rested upon public opinion, and they corresponded to contemporary psychiatric thought and reflected Polish legal tradition. While there was a consensus about the need to protect individual rights of mentally disturbed persons legally via the courts, some concern was expressed that the Proposal's criteria for involuntary commitment needed to be narrowed further.

Discussions of the Draft Proposal within psychiatric circles generally occurred at meetings sponsored by regional chapters of the Polish Psychiatric Association. At each of these meetings a member of the Expert Commission — either an attorney or a psychiatrist — attended each of these meetings. As expected, the matter of the Proposal generated heated debate, for, depending upon the psychiatric tradition of a given region and the orientation of its professionals, the Proposal was viewed either as an infringement upon the traditional autonomy of the Polish psychiatric practitioner, or as a much-needed reorganization of the entire psychiatric service delivery system consonant with contemporary thought. These discussions clearly revealed that a large majority of psychiatric practitioners had not given much consideration to the social and legal aspects of the doctor-patient relationship. Furthermore, many psychiatrists tended to administer treatment without the patient's consent, fully believing such decisions to be within the legitimate scope of medical discretion. It was widely believed, for example, that a patient's need for involuntary treatment was purely a matter of the physician's personal judgment. It is noteworthy that the major opposition to the legal regulation of mental health, or to the basic assumptions of "The Theses," was limited to a handful of articles, all written by older psychiatrists.

Some discussants openly supported the Proposal either totally or with minor modifications. They expressed some question about the need to restructure the overall mental health care delivery system and about the grounds for involuntary commitment which were so narrow that they failed to cover many situations requiring involuntary treatment encountered in practice. A fear was also expressed that the great number of cases which would be referred to the Court under the Proposal might impair the Court's effectiveness in adjudicating mental health matters.

Whatever else, the far-reaching scope and fervor of the discussions provided clear evidence that the Draft Proposal had addressed a critical social need and that it brought to the surface painful problems, heretofore hidden or shrouded under the mantle of medical discretion, which now required clarification and legal regulation.[3] The Commission of Experts agreed with the public that pas-

[3]S. Dabrowski, "Informacja o projekcie ustawy o ochronie zdrowia psychicznego," *Psychiatr. Pol.* 1 (1976): 65–74.

sage of the Draft Proposal could no longer be postponed, for the existing legal gap regarding such matters as involuntary treatment had led to harmful misunderstandingo which, because of their significance to society as a whole, made more visible and legal regulation imperative.

The discussions had also confirmed the need for a comprehensive Mental Health Act which would encompass the totality of mental health issues in Poland, and, in so doing, would take existing socio-cultural and legal imperatives fully into account.

Poland's Existing Mental Health System

The need for comprehensive legislation is clearly demonstrated by the expanding demand for mental health services, the extent to which those demands are not being met qualitatively or quantitatively, and the lack of legal regulations for certain mental health services.

The steadily increasing rate in the reported incidence and prevalence of mental disturbance in Poland supports the demand for more and better mental health care. As of 1976, the prevalence of mental disturbances (excluding alcoholic disturbances) reported by out-patient facilities was 1,407 per 100,000 population with a corresponding incidence of 454 per 100,000. The admission rate, as reported by all inpatient facilities, was 380 per 100,000 with first admissions accounting for less than 50% of all admissions. The total number of inpatients as of the end of 1975 was over 37,000, the average length of stay being 83 days. Given this epidemiological situation as well as developmental trends observed worldwide, it seems reasonable to expect a further expansion of psychiatric disturbances in Poland, well beyond that which could be expected from a general population increase.

Currently, psychiatric care in Poland is administered within the general health service system and consists of: (a) a relatively tight, though still incomplete network of outpatient psychiatric clinics (over 460 units) and outpatient units for alcoholic patients (over 430 units) incorporated within Local Health Centers; (b) a very loose network of badly-distributed, large and mid-sized mental hospitals, none of which is secure (45 units), psychiatric departments in general hospitals (22 units), and inpatient units for alcoholic patients (8 units); (c) very few day hospitals (33 units) and domiciliary care facilities (2 units); (d) shelter workshops for mental and severely mentally retarded patients (120 units for 55 hundred patients); and (e) nursing homes (208 units) for 25,000 chronic mental and severely mentally retarded patients.[4]

According to general health service rules, outpatient and inpatient units as well as most psychiatric hospital wards and psychiatric units in general hospitals are linked to catchment areas. Hospital psychiatric ward teams are functionally and administratively integrated with outpatient teams covering the same catchment area.

Primary health care facilities also deliver services to mentally disturbed indi-

---

[4]T. Dziduszko and S. Dabrowski, "Rozwoj psychiatrycznej opieki zdrowotnej w. Polsce," *Psychiatr. Pol.* 6 (1974): 631—648.

viduals, particularly those with neurotic disorders. In fact, 71 percent of all psychiatric services are delivered by primary care units.[5]

The activities of local inpatient and outpatient psychiatric care facilities are professionally reviewed and supervised by provincial and regional specialists appointed by the Minister of Health and Social Welfare. Psychiatric departments of medical academies also may be vested with regional supervisory responsibilities while psychiatric standards at a national level are defined by a Professional Advisory Board. The Psychoneurological Institute in Warsaw constitutes the executive body of this Board. Supervising personnel also investigate and, if possible, resolve patients' complaints filed with local authorities or directly with the Ministry of Health and Social Welfare.

Existing legislation regulates psychiatric interventions in criminal cases (Criminal Code, Code of Criminal Proceedings), in civil cases (Civil Code, Code of Civil Proceedings) and in cases relating to family and guardianship matters (Family and Guardianship Code). The involuntary treatment of alcoholics also is legally regulated (Antialcoholic Law). In accordance with this law, a person may be subjected to involuntary treatment if he or she manifests symptoms of chronic alcoholism resulting in a serious breakdown of family relationships, demoralization of minors, dangerousness to others, or continued disruptions of the public order. The required proceedings are initiated by a special commission for involuntary alcoholic treatment, the involuntary commitment to a mental hospital or alcoholic inpatient facility being adjudicated by the District Court in nonadversary proceeding. Involuntary commitment of mentally disturbed persons, in contrast, has not yet been regulated by Polish law. Instead, it is based on a Directive of the Ministry of Health and Social Welfare established in 1952.

The Promotion of Mental Health Envisioned by the Draft Proposal

A primary assumption of the Draft Proposal is that mental health is conceptually broader than mental health care and includes preventive services. The proposed legislation therefore does not limit itself merely to regulating the more troublesome aspects of the doctor-patient relationship, but rather addresses the fundamental tasks of insuring mental health.

These tasks, as enumerated in the Draft Proposal, include: (a) creating conditions favorable to the promotion of good mental health in areas such as the growth and development of children, schooling, family life, work and leisure, and other aspects of life in the society, while combating adverse influences in these areas; (b) providing mentally disturbed individuals with comprehensive, accessible health services as well as with other forms of care and assistance essential for living in the social environment; and (c) promoting principles of mental health and fostering positive social attitudes toward the mentally disturbed.

It seems obvious that the implementation of such broadly defined functions goes far beyond the traditional functions of the Ministry of Health and Social Welfare. Thus the Draft Proposal requires that state and local government

[5]K. Zukowska and T. Dziduszko, "Udział podstawowej opieki zdrowotnej w swiadczeniach dla osob z zaburzeniami psychicznymi," (in press).

authorities in conjunction with various other institutions implement its mandates within the context of fulfilling their obligations. Social organizations and luual tenanto' oouncils[6] also operate as active participants in accomplishing mental health goals.

To insure that its mandates will be carried out effectively, the Draft Proposal establishes a central advisory and consultative body, the Mental Health Council, which is directly responsible to the Prime Minister. In addition to its advisory and consultative functions, the Council is also charged with designing programs to meet mental health objectives within a broadly-defined preventive framework. A substantial part of these programs, however, would be carried out by local councils of community residents.

The second major task contemplated by the Draft Proposal seeks to answer a question, namely, how can mentally disturbed individuals be provided the health care services and assistance they need to maintain themselves in their social milieu? The Drafts Proposal's answer to this question may be found in its provisions in two specific areas: (a) psychiatric health care for mentally disturbed individuals, and (b) a wide range of supportive social welfare, nursing, and educational services.

Primary health care facilities, along with specialized psychiatric institutions, would be required to provide services such as emergency assistance, outpatient care, partial or home hospitalization, and full hospitalization. A broad social-protective-educational base for these services would, in turn, be provided by many existing or proposed institutions and offices. Thus a most significant role would be played by existing social welfare residence homes, sheltered workshop facilities, and subsidized work settings, while additional assistance could be provided by proposed facilities including day centers for occupational rehabilitation purposes, special residence homes, and hostels.

The model being presented by the Draft Proposal would, if enacted, fulfill several important functions. It would ensure the integration of psychiatric health care within the broader complex of social welfare-nursing-educational services. The model would also foster the evolution of urgently-needed rehabilitative and social welfare facilities. And it would establish a framework encompassing legal regulations for providing differential health care and social welfare services. Most importantly, the Draft Proposal's model provides a basis for transforming traditional concepts of outpatient and inpatient psychiatric care into new approaches which are expected to be both effective and economical.

Treatment, Rehabilitation, Care and Assistance under the Draft Proposal

A separate chapter of the Draft Proposal is addressed to general principles regarding the examination, treatment and rehabilitation of mentally disturbed individuals. These principles define the legal contours of the physician-patient relationship in order to safeguard the constitutional rights of individuals as well as the ethical mandates of the medical profession. These principles require expression in a mental health act because, even though they are commonly ob-

---

[6]B. Hernacka and T. Zakowska-Dabrowska, "Postepowanie lekarskie w chwili przyjecia a stosunek chorych do hospitalizacji psychiatrycznej," *Psychiatr. Pol.* 3 (1975): 263–265.

served for medical patients generally, their applicability to mentally disturbed individuals has apparently been questioned in actual practice and in psychiatric hospitals where they have often been ignored. These principles include:

1. *The Principle of Self-Determination* which requires the patient's (or his legal representative's) consent for all examinations, treatments, rehabilitation, and care. Specific consent is required for certain types of treatment such as surgical operations or other therapeutic modalities known to entail an above-average risk. The Draft Proposal does allow, in emergency situations, the administration of treatment that is essential to save a patient's life.

2. *The Principle of Informed Consent* is an essential complement of the preceding principle. The physician is therefore required to inform the patient (and/or his legal representative) about the purpose and expected results of any therapeutic procedure. The Draft Proposal, however, does foresee the possibility of exempting the physician from any responsibility to convey such information if that action could have antitherapeutic consequences for the patient.

3. *The Principle of Free Contact and Correspondence* assures the patient a right to communicate with his family and others. The written correspondence of patients is therefore exempt from hospital censorship.

4. *The Principle of Respect for the Whole of a Patient's Needs* (within the treatment process) provides that health goals cannot be reached at all costs, for instance, at the expense of other personal (e.g., moral, intellectual and professional) needs of the patient.

The remaining principles within the Draft Proposal relate to rehabilitative activities and payment to patients for work which they perform. Rehabilitative activities carried out within psychiatric facilities, for example, constitute an integral part of the treatment program and thus cannot be undertaken merely in response to economic considerations. When patients do perform work on behalf of psychiatric facilities, they must be compensated according to prevailing standards elsewhere in the economy.

The Draft Proposal also establishes the general contours of community-based care to be afforded those who, because of mental disturbance, are not able to meet their own basic needs without outside assistance. Such care seeks to assure individuals assistance in resolving problems in living in their social environment as well as in meeting their basic material and socio-cultural needs.

In relation to the Principle of Self-Determination in regard to treatment, a difficult problem arises in psychiatric practice concerning the "consent" given by a patient who, as a result of mental disturbance, is not capable of self-determination. Informed consent cannot be defective if it is to be legally valid. According to Article 82 of the Polish Civil Code, a declaration made by one who is not fully capable of making decisions and freely expressing his will is invalid. Consequently, how can one regard as valid "consent" a statement which, according to the Civil Code, is legally worthless? To resolve this problem by resort to competency proceedings would create bureaucratic obstacles which would further hinder admission of the patient to a psychiatric facility and delay his treatment. For certain patients, especially those with transient mental disturbances, a legal finding of incompetency would also be undesirable insofar as the patient's total and continued personal welfare is concerned. Moreover, authorizing the patient's actual caretaker to give consent to his hospitalization would be a questionable procedure because a caretaker's motives and decisions may not comport with the patient's interests. Regulations are needed on the one hand to eliminate practices which are at odds with the Civil Code and, on the other hand, to free physicians to administer necessary treatment even when the patient is not able to give valid consent for such treatment.

"The Theses" which were first submitted for public debate sought to resolve this dilemma by requiring the hospital to notify the Guardianship Court whenever a voluntarily admitted patient was not capable, at the time of admission, of giving valid consent. Such a notification would have enabled the Court to issue necessary instructions regarding hospitalization and treatment.

In response to many questions which were raised in discussions concerning that provision, it was decided to replace the Civil Code's formulation of a "conscious and free expression of one's will" with the criterion of an ability to recognize the *place* and the *purpose* of hospitalization. The new provision now reads: "If the mentally disturbed or mentally retarded person does not protest against admission, but is unable to understand where he is or why he was brought there, the admitting facility shall notify the Guardianship Court within 48 hours of admission, so as to secure the necessary instructions." This new criterion thus defines more realistically the category of patients whose consent for admission is considered defective.

In response to doubts about the results of implementing this change it was decided to try it during actual admissions. In particular, the researchers hoped to uncover any significant diversity of interpreting the standard, as well as to determine how frequently patients, at the time of admission, could not recognize "the place or purpose of hospitalization." Establishing the incidence of such cases would help in estimating the extent to which the Guardianship Court would be burdened with new responsibilities.[7]

The research, involving 1,600 admissions in nine mental hospitals, showed that the majority (65%) of patients at the time of admission give consent and that the consent given by a decisive majority of those patients was legally valid. Patients who would have been referred to the court because of their inability to give valid consent ranged from 1.6 to 4.5 percent of all admissions. An inability to offer legally valid consent most often occurred among patients whose mental disturbance was organically caused.

Involuntary Treatment Under the Draft Proposal

Involuntary examination, treatment and detention in a psychiatric facility are seen as serious departures from the Principle of Self-Determination and

[7]S. Dabrowski, K. Gerard, S. Walczak, B. Woronowicz, and T. Zakowska, "Brak zdolnosci do wyrazania zgody na przyjecie i leczenie w zamknietym zakladzie psychiatrycznej opieki zdrowotnej," (in press).

such procedures are therefore regulated with great care. The Draft Proposal defines quite precisely the requirements for proceeding against the patient's will, limiting such actions to cases in which all three of the following criteria are met: (a) the presence of a mental disturbance; (b) the manifestation of specific behaviors which indicate that a direct threat to the patient's own life or to the life or health of others is either already present, or is likely to develop in the near future; and (c) the threat to self or others is caused by the patient's existing mental disturbance. "Mental disturbance" is broadly defined to include not only mental disease, namely the psychoses and mental retardation, but also neurotic disturbances and personality disorders.

The need to define the requisite criteria narrowly results from the necessity to respect the autonomy of the individual as well as from an appreciation of the therapeutic imperative which holds, generally speaking, that consent for treatment is a fundamental prerequisite for its effectiveness. It is self-evident that a psychiatric examination, on an outpatient basis where possible, is essential to determine the need for involuntary hospitalization and treatment. The Draft Proposal permits such an examination without the consent of the person involved when it is established via the direct testimony of third parties, interviews conducted in the person's own community, and the personal conclusions of physicians that the individual's behavior confirms the presence of the three stated criteria for involuntary hospitalization. In order to remove an immediate threat to the health or life of either the person involved or others, a physician is allowed to initiate indispensable therapeutic procedures and, if necessary, to use physical restraints.

A central feature of any mental health act concerns its provisions for involuntary hospitalization. The "Theses" noted earlier provided for two categories of involuntary commitment. The second category, however, was significantly changed in the current Draft Proposal as the result of discussions occasioned by the "Theses." The first category permitting involuntary commitment occurs only when the individual's prior behavior indicates that, as a result of his mental disturbance, he presents a direct threat to his own life or to the life or health of others. Once the examining physician has confirmed the three commitment prerequisites, the patient may be immediately hospitalized. The director of the admitting facility is required to notify the Guardianship Court within 48 hours of the patient's involuntary admission and the Court, in turn, is required to hear the matter without cost to the patient within 14 days of such notification. Whether or not the patient is to be civilly committed is determined by a judge and two assessors (citizen-magistrates) after the patient and two expert witnesses, both psychiatrists, have been heard. The physician who took part in the decision to admit the patient against his will, or to deny his request for discharge, can not appear as an expert witness. Also, the patient must be represented by an attorney. The Court may order the hearing to be conducted in the patient's psychiatric facility, and the proceeding may be closed to the public at the patient's request. The patient has a right to be present at the hearing and to have access to all testimony presented. The Court may terminate the proceeding if the patient voluntarily agrees to continued hospitalization. Before dismissing the proceedings, however, the Judge is required to listen to the patient in order to verify that his consent to stay in the hospital has been given voluntarily. This requirement is waived if the patient has already been discharged from the treatment institution.

The provisions encompassed by this category of involuntary commitments closely resemble current practices stemming from the 1952 Directive of the Ministry of Health and Social Welfare. These administrative directives allow psychiatric hospitalizations of individuals at their own request, or at the request of a relative, legal representative, or actual caretaker. The Court (or the district attorney) is also authorized to order such a course of action. An admitting physician can order emergency commitment only in those cases in which delay would either have a strongly adverse effect on the patient's condition, or would endanger the life of the patient or others. Such an order may be implemented immediately, and is, at least theoretically, not subject to appeal. In practice, an appeal is occasionally made to the director of the hospital, the Court, the district attorney, the Department of Health, the Ministry of Health and Social Welfare, or the Psychoneurological Institute in Warsaw. There exists no general policy for responding to such appeals, however.

The second category of involuntary commitment under the Draft Proposal predicates admission to the hospital upon an order of the Guardianship Court based upon a petition filed by the patient's spouse, a blood relative, or actual caretaker. The only basis for such involuntary admission must be the *legal* determination that the prior behavior of the proposed patient indicates that he is mentally disturbed and that, without inpatient treatment, he will, in the near future, threaten his own life or the life or health of others. The petition for involuntary hospitalization under this provision must be accompanied by the supporting opinion of a psychiatrist on staff of the psychiatric outpatient clinic covering the region of the proposed patient's residence or stay. The composition of the Court and the procedure utilized are the same as previously indicated for the first category. The decision of the District Guardian Court, though appealable (by either the proposed patient or the petitioner) to the Provincial Court, is immediately enforced.

Although the second category broadens the basis for involuntary commitment beyond the presence of a direct threat, it provides special requirements which serve to safeguard the rights of the individual. The authors of the Draft Proposal are well aware that predicting dangerousness is a very difficult matter and that psychiatrists have not always proved themselves to be the best experts in this matter.[8, 9, 10] It appears, however, that given the absence of the second category of involuntary commitment, Polish psychiatrists would have tended to interpret the first category so broadly as to include the second. Such an outcome might well have been more unfortunate than the potential tendency to overpredict dangerousness insofar as the second category is concerned. Thus it was the explicit mandate of the Expert Commission that the final decision in commitments of the second category be made by the Court.

[8]A. M. Dershowitz, "The Psychiatrist's Power in Civil Commitment," *Psychology Today* Feb. 1969, pp. 43–47.

[9]A. Rosen, "Detection of Suicidal Patients: An Example of Some Limitations in the Prediction of Infrequent Events," *Journal of Consulting Psychology* 18 (1954): 397–403.

[10]S. A. Shah, "Dangerousness and Civil Commitment of the Mentally Ill: Some Public Policy Considerations," *American Journal of Psychology* 5 (1975): 509–505.

The Draft Proposal holds that the involuntarily admitted patient may be given, with or without his consent, necessary medical treatments, but that the patient's consent will be required for surgical operations and treatment modalities entailing an above-average risk. The use of physical restraints is limited to those situations in which they are essential to the administration of necessary medical procedures and when less intrusive means would prove ineffective.

The decision to discharge a patient does not require court approval, but is made by the chief of the ward in which the patient is being treated. Once it is confirmed that the legal prerequisites for involuntary hospitalization no longer exist, the patient has been discharged. The Guardianship Court is notified when an involuntary patient is discharged. The request for discharge from inpatient psychiatric care may be made by the involuntary patient himself, his legal representative, spouse, blood relative, or guardian. The request may not be filed earlier than 30 days after the Guardianship Court ordered involuntary admission (or further involuntary detention) in the inpatient facility.

. The Principle of Self-Determination applies equally in regard to the placement of mentally disturbed or mentally retarded individuals in need of continued care and nursing services outside a hospital setting. In those exceptional situations, when the person involved refuses to give consent for the placement even though such placement may be essential for his survival, the matter is adjudicated by the Guardianship Court at the request of the local department of state administration.

The responsibility of legal authorities vis-à-vis involuntary commitment should be seen as one of the most important issues to be resolved by any Polish mental health legislation which is finally adopted into law. Entrusting the Guardianship Courts with jurisdiction over such cases is in harmony with the traditional principle in Polish law that any deprivation of freedom must be closely monitored by the Courts. If the Courts maintain control over decisions regarding the deprivation of freedom for those who have violated the legal order as well as those who, because of their alcoholism, are subjected to involuntary treatment, it would appear imperative that court supervision and legal principles should apply to those who are to be deprived of their freedom because of dangerousness induced by their mental disturbance. Actually the reason for involuntary hospitalization and treatment should be the welfare of such patients. Nevertheless, patients are likely to perceive such an experience as a deprivation of their freedom. Placing these matters under the jurisdiction of the Court seems guaranteed to enhance public confidence that the civil rights of individuals are being recognized and respected. The Court's involvement also has additional advantages insofar as extending the applicability of the Code of Civil Procedure to mental health matters does not require a special adjudicatory procedure yet lends support to the uniformity of existing Polish law.

The Draft Proposal also requires the Guardianship Court, in addition to its aforementioned functions, to oversee the provision of community-based care, and to visit facilities which house mentally disturbed individuals and interview patients who have been there for six months or longer.

During the wide-ranging public discussion of the Draft Proposal referred to earlier, some critics of the proposed legislation contended that if the Drafts were enacted into law, the legal responsibilities thereby thrust upon psychiatrists would take too much time from their regular clinical duties. Furthermore, they claimed that the courts would either be unable to process the flood of cases or that the strain exerted on the courts would substantially lower the quality and effectiveness of their adjudications of mental health matters. These predictions seemed to be based on cursory observations of prevailing admission practices. Thus, one unpublished report on a Warsaw area hospital claimed that the percentage of involuntary patients was approximately 50%. However, carefully designed research has found such figures to be seriously inflated. Studies published by the Poznan Psychiatric Department of Medical Academy show that only 7.1% of all admissions were clearly involuntary while an equal number of patients were, at the moment of their admission, unable because of disorientation or lack of contact with their surroundings to make a decision regarding hospitalization.[11, 12] When the procedure was experimentally changed to require patients to give written consent to their hospitalization, the number of those refusals to give such consent rose to 11%.[13]

In order to clarify these divergent findings, the admissions to nine large psychiatric hospitals were carefully studied.[14] The research utilized a questionnaire, filled out by physicians at the time of admission and one week thereafter in which the following information, along with other data, was obtained: (a) the patient's ability to recognize the place and purpose of hospitalization; (b) the patient's reaction to hospitalization (consent or protest); and (c) the presence or absence of the patient's direct threat to self or others.

An analysis of findings based upon a total of 1,628 admissions revealed that enactment of the Draft Proposal would not place a heavy burden either upon psychiatrists, as expert witnesses, or upon the Guardianship Court itself. The number of reported involuntary admissions varied widely, ranging from 3 to 38 percent (25% on the average). The hospitals with a high percentage of involuntary admissions did not report a correspondingly high percentage of patients presenting a threat to themselves or others. This might well indicate that higher percentages of involuntary admissions are not based as much upon the condition of the patients, as reflected by their dangerousness, as upon subjective attitudes of the examining physicians. Such attitudes, already clearly evident in earlier discussions, are based upon a tendency to extend the grounds for involuntary admission far beyond the limits of direct threat to one's own life or to the life or health of others.

The findings further reveal that the *minimum* percentage of patients referred to the Guardianship Court to determine their need for involuntary hospitalization is about 20.6%, the maximum constituting approximately 33.9% of all admissions. The difference between the two figures is based upon the number of "difficult to establish" responses. The minimum percentage of all patients admitted who would come to the attention of the Guardianship Court for deter-

[11] B. Hernacka and T. Zakowska-Dabrowska, "Czynniki wplywajace na stosunek pacjenta do hospitalizacji psychiatrycznej," *Psychiatr. Pol.* 3 (1973): 299–304.

[12] B. Hernacka and T. Zakowska-Dabrowska, "Dobrowolnosc i przymus hospitalizacji psychiatrycznej w swietle materialow Kliniki Psychiatrycznej AM w Poznaniu," *Psychiatr. Pol.* 2 (1973): 195–196.

[13] B. Hernacka and Zakowska-Dabrowska, "Postepowanie lekarskie w chwili przyjecia a stosunek chorych do hospitalizacji psychiatrycznej," *Psychiatr. Pol.* 3 (1975): 263–265.

[14] B. Hernacka and T. Zakowska-Dabrowska, "Dobrowolnosc i przymus hospitalizacji psychiatrycznej

mination of the need for involuntary hospitalization and treatment (after deducting cases in which proceedings would be terminated as the result of the patient volunteering consent to treatment prior to a court hearing) approximates 11.4%, the maximum being 19.6%. The total percentage of court cases resulting from the new legislation would therefore apparently constitute only about 1.9% of all civil cases and 5.6% of all nonadversary cases. There are some indications that even these percentages will, in all probability, prove to be inflated.

Conclusion

The limited scope of this paper does not allow the presentation of all issues which are encompassed by the Draft Proposal. Some important topics, as well as a comparison with corresponding regulations in other countries, have been omitted out of necessity.

The Draft Proposal is a comprehensive document addressed to state and local government authorities, to social organizations, to local councils of community residents and to a number of medical and nonmedical specialists. It is, nevertheless, primarily addressed to psychiatrists upon whom the actual realization of its thrust will be heavily dependent. Recalling the attitudes of some senior psychiatrists during the discussion phase of the Draft Proposal, the internalization and adoption of such legislation will not be an easy matter. Regardless of foreseen difficulties, the fact is that the process of adoption has already begun. This is expressed by an ever-increasing tendency in Poland to limit the grounds for involuntary commitment, to extend the rights of patients, and to modernize hospital practices. A recent article in a Warsaw newspaper catches the spirit of these changes. The reporter, in describing the difficulties in hospitalizing a non-dangerous psychiatric patient, concludes that "the proposed Mental Health Act has begun to be observed by psychiatrists even before being passed by the Sejm." If other elements of the Draft Proposal succeed in occasioning similar motivational and educational recognitions, we can well expect that the essence of the proposed legislation will find ultimate expression and social recognition.

Comments on Dabrowski's "Major Issues in the Polish Mental Health Legislation Draft Proposal"

Commentator: P. Browning Hoffman*

We are most indebted to Dr. Dabrowski for an authoritative appraisal of Poland's Mental Health Legislation Draft Proposal[1] which was created by the 1974 Commission of Experts which he chaired. Perhaps in his modesty Dr. Dabrowski has failed to convey the importance of that Proposal, for if ultimately enacted, it will replace the only existing Polish regulation governing hospitalization of the mentally ill, namely a 1952 Directive of the Ministry of Health and Social Welfare.[2] The Directive does not distinguish between voluntary and involuntary psychiatric treatment and permits relatives, guardians or physicians to hospitalize patients deemed dangerous to themselves and/or others with no legal mechanism by which to appeal such decisions.

The Draft Proposal described by Dr. Dabrowski is a unique departure from Polish tradition for other reasons as well. Increasingly since World War II, the Polish people have expressed trust in their judiciary as well as interest in the psychiatric care afforded their mentally ill countrymen. By 1970 pressure for legislative reform of Poland's mental health code had crystallized in proposed legislation which distinguished between voluntary and involuntary psychiatric treatment, but which left the administration of all forms of treatment largely within the discretion of the psychiatric profession and thus beyond judicial scrutiny.[3] Indeed, the 1970 proposal was submitted to the Polish legislature secretly, without opportunity for public review and debate. When finally exposed, public outrage prompted its immediate withdrawal from further legislative consideration. The Draft Proposal which is under discussion today constitutes the fifteenth attempt to enact legislation in Poland to replace the 26-year-old Directive of the Ministry of Health and Social Welfare.

Many provisions of the Polish Draft Proposal are progressive compared with prevailing standards in other countries. The provision that all voluntary patients

*Professor of Law and Psychiatry, University of Virginia, Charlottsville, Virginia 22901 (USA).

This commentary is based upon two drafts of Dr. Stanislaw Dabrowski's article and upon various interpretations of the Proposed Polish Mental Health Act (or "Draft Proposal") as it has evolved under the guidance of the 1974 Commission of Experts. These realities, plus the exigencies of translating Polish documents into English accurately, may account for certain misunderstandings concerning the Draft Proposal's minor provisions, but not its basic thrust.

[1]S. Dabrowski, "Major Issues in the Polish Mental Health Legislation Draft Proposal," *Int. J. Law and Psychiatry* 1 (1978): 125–136.

[2]Polish Ministry of Health and Social Welfare Directive #120/52, Dec. 10, 1952.

[3]L. L. Frydman, "Psychiatric Hospitalization in Poland: An Overview and Some Comparisons," unpublished manuscript, Jan. 22, 1977.

must affirmatively "consent" to hospitalization by stating the place and the purpose of their treatment has no parallel in the United States where non-protesting, but often ambivalent patients are assumed to consent to treatment merely by virtue of their acquiescence to hospitalization. The same may be said for the requirement that two independent psychiatrists attend Polish civil commitment proceedings in order to review evidence and provide assistance to the court. The Polish Draft Proposal is also unique in requiring judges who conduct guardianship and civil commitment proceedings to visit and even monitor the facilities which receive their charges. Finally, the Draft Proposal's evolution by heated public debate and its emphasis upon the broad integration of mental health resources at a community level illustrate an unusual public interest in the care afforded mentally disturbed persons.

Undeniably, the Draft Proposal signifies Poland's willingness to enact major legislative reforms in the area of mental health. Similar reforms have been attempted in other countries including the United States. Poland now shares a basic dilemma with those countries: how is enlightened legislation to be translated into actual practice? The Draft Proposal presently contains several ambiguous provisions which would appear to frustrate that critical transition. The purpose of this commentary is to question some of those provisions and to anticipate certain future problems in light of United States experiences with similar legislation.

1. Ambiguities in the Polish Draft Proposal

"Voluntary"Psychiatric Hospitalization

Relying upon the "Principle of Self-Determination," the Draft Proposal predicates voluntary psychiatric treatment of legally competent adults upon their consent to undergo such treatment.[4] Under a similar legal prerequisite for voluntary care in the United States, the *truly* voluntary patient would also request — or consent to — treatment.

Unfortunately, a substantial number of mentally ill persons neither seek nor reject treatment by visibly offering or withholding consent. These patients, when faced with the prospect of psychiatric hospitalization, choose not to protest the circumstances of their treatment essentially for two different reasons: either they really do not care what happens to them, or they perceive that they will be legally committed to treatment against their will if they protest, and they acquiesce to treatment in order to avoid that legal proceeding. Whatever the rationale, the "non-protesting" patient is not a truly voluntary patient. Moreover, the "non-protesting" patient is not distinguished from the truly voluntary patient either within U.S. civil commitment codes or during the legal proceedings which they authorize. Therefore, U.S. patients who choose hospitalization in order to avoid the stigma and trauma of formal commitment proceedings are technically classified as "voluntary," while their counterparts who evidence no interest whatsoever in the circumstances of their care may receive,

---

[4]Proposed Polish Mental Health Act ["Draft Proposal"], Article 16(#1), Article 17, Article 22(#1), Article 28(#1), Article 32(#1) and Article 40(#2), (unpublished) 1978.

at best, clinical designations such as "apathetic," "isolated," "autistic," etc. Insofar as there is no difference in the treatment afforded voluntary and involuntary patients within the hospital, there may be no need to distinguish between truly voluntary, "non-protesting" and involuntary patients. But these distinctions may be critical insofar as the three types of patients receive differential care, especially to the extent that a patient's status at the time of admission implies something about his competency to accept or refuse treatment.

Under Poland's Draft Proposal, the voluntary patient must request or consent to care by stating the purpose and place of treatment. The consent required by the Draft Proposal does not meet a legal standard of *informed* consent for psychiatric treatment, however. Informed consent requires (a) knowledge of one's condition and its treatment(s); (b) competence to weigh treatment alternatives and indicate a choice; and (c) sufficient freedom to make a voluntary choice.[5] If one assumes that the majority of acutely ill psychiatric patients who require hospitalization are not capable of giving informed consent for such interventions, the Draft Proposal's lesser standard of consent may be entirely appropriate. But how does the Draft Proposal's consent standard distinguish non-protesting from truly voluntary patients? The patient who simply does not care about the circumstances of his treatment or the patient who would protest his hospitalization if not threatened with a commitment proceeding would seem as able – and perhaps as likely – to know the place and purpose of treatment as the truly voluntary patient. Or, in the alternative, does the Draft Proposal imply that distinctions between voluntary and non-protesting patients are either immaterial, illogical or both?[6]

Of course, one important theoretical advantage may be gained by requiring even a minimal standard of consent for voluntary hospitalization. The patient in Poland who lacks the ability (competency) to state even the "place and purpose" of treatment thereby triggers a specific determination of his competency by the Guardianship Court which may then offer certain "instructions" concerning his further treatment.[7] It is unclear, however, what procedural devices and standards of competency are utilized by the Guardianship Court in deriving such instructions.

"Involuntary" Psychiatric Treatment

The most critical questions raised by Poland's Draft Proposal concern its justifications and procedures for involuntary psychiatric treatment. These ques-

---

[5] P. B. Hoffman, "The Right to Refuse Psychiatric Treatment: A Clinical Perspective," *Bull. Amer. Acad. Psychiat. and Law.* 5 (1977): 295.

[6] If so, it is interesting to note what happened when Polish psychiatric patients were required to consent to hospitalization in writing in order to be classified as "voluntary" admissions. As reported by the Poenan Department of Psychiatry of the Polish Academy of Medicine, requiring the patient's written consent for voluntary hospitalization led to almost a 4% increase in the number of *in*voluntary admissions. While many explanations might be offered to account for this result, one interpretation would be that non-protesting (but ambivalent) patients, once aware that they can oppose hospitalization by withholding written consent, prefer to exercise a right to refuse treatment rather than accept what is offered in silence. See B. Hernacka and T. Zakowska-Dabrowska, "Postepowanie Lekarskie w Chevili Przyjecia a Stosunek Chorych do Hospitalizacji Psychiatrycznej," *Psychiat. Pol.,* 3 (1975): 263–265.

[7] Proposed Polish Mental Health Act ["Draft Proposal"], Article 29, (unpublished) 1978.

tions are not unique to Poland, for they arise within virtually any legislation which permits involuntary psychiatric care. The ultimate success or failure of the Draft Proposal, however, may well depend upon its effectiveness in dealing with involuntary patients.

Under provisions of the Draft Proposal, involuntary psychiatric treatment would be warranted upon (a) the existence of "mental disturbance" for the patient; (b) his apparent dangerousness to himself and/or others, and (c) his inability to seek treatment voluntarily.[8]

It is important to recognize that "mental disturbance" includes, *inter alia*, "either chronic or transient deviations in psychic functioning," but not psychoneuroses and personality disorders.[9] Given Frydman's assertion that Polish psychiatric hospitals treat only psychotic disorders for the most part, "mental disturbance," despite its broad definition, may operate in practice to limit involuntary hospitalizations to those patients who exhibit acute, florid and disabling psychotic symptoms.[10] Unfortunately, however, the Draft Proposal's language may be broad enough to permit involuntary treatment of non-psychotic persons whose lifestyles, while self-sufficient, could be considered socially annoying, bizarre, or even politically dissident. Surely the potential for such abuse, as manifested in other countries,[11] warrants defining more visible criteria for mental disturbances which, by their severity, justify involuntary psychiatric treatment.

The Polish Draft Proposal, like U.S. civil commitment codes which rely upon the patient's presumed dangerousness as a justification for involuntary treatment, raises question as to the definition, let alone the predictability, of that elusive characteristic.[12] In emphasizing "specific behavior" which constitutes a "direct threat" to one's self or another, the Proposal attempts to narrow the concept of dangerousness to visible behaviors which might be regarded as dangerous by most persons. But must the "specific behavior" be an act of physical aggression, or will merely the threat of such an act suffice? How immediate must the act or threat be? The Draft Proposal, under one of its two civil commitment procedures, includes dangerous acts which are likely to occur "in the near future."[13] This emphasis upon potential as opposed to past "dangerousness" suggests further that a patient's status, without any previous "overt act," may suffice to meet the required standard of dangerousness. Finally, the Draft Proposal defines dangerousness in one section in terms of harm to property as well as harm to persons. How much harm to property must be demonstrated in

---

[8]The criteria for civil commitability are not so precisely defined in the current Draft Proposal. They are, however, intended to apply within the context of that document (personal communication with S. Dabrowski, Feb. 24, 1978) and were reflected in its earlier drafts. See W. Daszkiewicz, S. Dabrowski, and L. Kurbricki, "The Nation and the Law," *Bull.* (Poland) 8–9 (1974): 342–343.

[9]Daszkiewicz et al., *supra*, note 8, p. 5 (trans. L. L. Frydman).

[10]L. L. Frydman, *supra*, note 3, p. 18.

[11]S. Bloch and P. Reddaway, *Psychiatric Terror* (New York: Basic Books, 1977).

[12]American Psychiatric Association, "Clinical Aspects of the Violent Individual," Task Force Report No. 8, 1974. See also J. Cocozza and H. Steadman, "The Failure of Psychiatric Predictions of Dangerousness: Clear and Convincing Evidence," *Rutgers Law Review,* 29 (1976): 1094–1098 and B. Diamond, "The Psychiatric Prediction of Dangerousness," *Univ. of Penn. Law Review* 123 (1974): 451–452.

[13]Proposed Polish Mental Health Act ["Draft Proposal"], Article 36(#1), (unpublished) 1978.

order to meet the dangerousness standard and, again, must the harm have occurred or merely be potential?

The Draft Proposal stipulates that the patient's impaired capacity to seek treatment voluntarily will serve as a justification for civil commitment. But how is this determination of incapacity to be made? Is the patient sufficiently impaired if he lacks the intellectual (if not emotional) capacity to perceive his illness and need for treatment as would a "rational man"? What about the dangerous patient who perceives his condition rationally, but prefers to go without treatment even at the cost of continued detention? Is he incompetent to the same extent or in the same way? It would be important to distinguish between these two patients if we desire to afford the first a trial of treatment and the second a right to refuse that trial.

Indeed, the precise contours of a patient's right to refuse treatment under the Draft Proposal are unclear. It would appear, for example, that patients may be treated against their will (i.e., without consent) in emergent circumstances or even following civil commitment unless the treatment is deemed hazardous and is thereby subject to scrutiny by the Guardianship Court or another external review agency. Like most U.S. civil commitment codes, "emergency" is vaguely defined and hazardous treatment can be so narrowly construed to vitiate any meaningful safeguard originally intended.

Presumably an involuntary patient could, as a practical matter, exercise a right to refuse treatment at any point during hospitalization, especially during judicial reviews to determine the need for further involuntary care. While the Draft Proposal provides for automatic judicial review at certain times, it does not state what alternative devices will be used to monitor the patient's progress at other times and throughout treatment. Nor does the Draft Proposal offer patients an expedient, non-legal mechanism to contest the circumstances of their care, a method to refuse even non-hazardous treatment if so desired. The monitoring of on-going (involuntary) psychiatric treatment and the methods by which patients may legitimately refuse treatment are of increasing concern to mental health professionals, judges, and legislators in the United States. As a result, numerous proposals have been made to allow patients the opportunities to request external reviews of their treatment programs by courts, administrative hearing officers,[14] legal aid attorneys,[15] patient advocates,[16] ombudsmen,[17] and

---

[14] This mechanism has been proposed in Pennsylvania and Michigan. See A. Halpern, "A Practicing Attorney Views the Right to Treatment," *Georgetown Law Journal,* 57 (1969): 782 [Pennsylvania proposal] and G. Morris, "Legal Problems Involved in Implementing the Right to Treatment," *Bull. Amer. Acad. of Psychiatry and Law* 1 (1973): 1 [Michigan Proposal].

[15] G. Morris, "Institutionalizing the Rights of Mental Patients: Committing the Legislature," *Cal. Law Review,* 62 (1974): 957.

[16] As authorized by the Virginia Legislature (Rights of Patients and Residents, Sec. 37.1-84.1, Va. Code Ann., 1976), The Commissioner of Mental Health and Mental Retardation has proposed "Regulations to Assure the Rights of Patients and Residents of [Virginia] Hospitals and Other Facilities." Lay patient advocates are to assume a major responsibility for protecting patients' rights in public sector facilities under terms of the Commissioner's Regulations. However, the Regulations have not yet been in effect long enough to evaluate their ultimate impact.

[17] Broderick, "A One-Legged Ombudsman in a Mental Hospital: An Over the Shoulder Glance at an Experimental Project," *Catholic Univ. Law Review,* 22 (1973): 517.

"treatment evaluators."[18] Does the Draft Proposal anticipate similar mechanisms to monitor involuntary psychiatric treatment? If so, what are their dimensions and limitations?

Although the Draft Proposal currently provides two separate, but conceptually related, procedures by which involuntary hospitalization may be carried out, neither seems to justify involuntary care upon a specific medicolegal determination that no less restrictive alternative to hospitalization will provide the patient with effective care. Many U.S. civil commitment codes require the court to determine that "no less restrictive alternative" to hospitalization will suffice to secure appropriate treatment for a patient. Without that finding, the court must either commit the patient to non-hospital treatment (where that disposition is allowed) or release the patient from any further judicial processing. While committing judges in at least one U.S. jurisdiction (Virginia) have expressed some confusion as to the precise legal meaning of a "least restrictive alternative" commitment requirement,[19] this is not to say that the concept itself is bad. The Draft Proposal could provide Poland with a unique opportunity to test the merits of a least restrictive alternative requirement.

2. Some Likely Problems

By way of concluding this brief commentary on the Polish Draft Proposal, I shall mention three general problems which may arise as the Proposal is implemented. For the most part, I base my concerns upon results which have obtained from attempting similar reforms in the United States.

First, I am awed by the sheer magnitude of the Draft Proposal's stated purpose — to promote good mental health "in areas such as the growth and development, child rearing, schooling, family life, work and leisure, and other aspects of life," to afford comprehensive mental health services which are "essential for living in the social environment," and to insure "proper social attitudes toward the mentally disturbed."[20]

I do not quarrel with the altruistic intentions expressed within these goals. But the Draft Proposal seems to authorize state supervision of virtually every aspect of life. I am hard pressed to define where the Proposal's therapeutic emphasis upon mental hygiene might end and its utilization for sociopolitical reform — possibly even oppressive reform — might begin. Moreover, on superficial analysis the Draft Proposal appears to grant mental health professionals an unusual degree of authority to define that boundary.

There are, perhaps, two other problems with the Draft Proposal's preference for the broad integration of mental health and social resources insofar as the goal is to be accomplished at a community level. On one hand, such community-based resources in the United States have often achieved disappointing results. They have not provided an economic panacea for the plight of many

[18]P. B. Hoffman and R. C. Dunn, "Beyond *Rouse* and *Wyatt*: An Administrative-Law Model for Expanding and Implementing the Mental Patient's Right to Treatment," *Virginia Law Review* 61 (1975): 297–339.

[19]P. B. Hoffman and L. L. Foust, "Least Restrictive Treatment of the Mentally Ill: A Doctrine in Search of its Senses," *San Diego Law Review,* 14 (1977): 1100–1154.

[20]Proposed Polish Mental Health Act ["Draft Proposal"], Article 2(#1), (unpublished) 1978.

mentally ill persons, but instead, in some cases, are both expensive and ineffi-
cient. On the other hand, community-based facilities are simply not appropriate for some psychiatric patients.[21] A number of states in the United States
have apparently forgotten this reality. In their enthusiasm for deinstitutionali-
zation, they have discharged many chronically disabled psychiatric patients
from the hospital only to see them suffer worse abuses within communities
which cannot — or will not — provide necessary assistance.[22]

The second problem which I foresee stems from the Draft Proposal's implicit
trust in legislative and judicial safeguards to prevent unwarranted or oppressive
psychiatric treatment. As the United States experience implies, the letter of the
law as expressed in mental health legislation may rarely be followed in practice,
particularly when insufficient financial resources are provided to accomplish
original legislative mandates. There is little evidence, in my opinion, that judicial safeguards function much better in assuring adequate treatment for mentally ill persons in the United States. Class action litigation seeking to change
entire mental health care delivery systems, for example, often destroys the
good as well as the bad within those systems. As a result, patients seeking relief suffer before, during and even after the litigation occurs.[23] Nor am I convinced that the elaborate "procedural due process" safeguards which often
govern civil commitment proceedings in the United States as well as under provisions of the Draft proposal actually have a beneficial impact. These are cosmetic efforts. They look good on paper, but they do not change the actual
practices of lawyers or mental health professionals. For example, the patient
facing a civil commitment proceeding is provided with an attorney. But that attorney is often torn between seeking what is perceived to be in the best interests of the client (e.g., hospitalization despite the client's wish for release) or
advocating the client's stated desire for release (despite a belief that immediate
release might further harm the client). With infrequent exceptions,[24] courts and
legislatures do not anticipate such dilemmas, let alone suggest methods for their
resolution.

My third concern seems tantamount to heresy given the obvious enthusiasm
within the Symposium on Law and Psychiatry and Poland's Proposed Mental
Health Legislation for multidisciplinary collaboration. It seems a popular as-

---

[21] F. Arnhoff, "Social Consequences of Policy Toward Mental Illness," *Science,* 188 (1974): 1277. See
also L. S. Kubie, "Pitfalls of Community Psychiatry," *Archives Gen. Psychiat.,* 18 (1968): 247.

[22] Reich and Siegel, "Psychiatry Under Siege: The Chronically Mentally Ill Shuffle to Oblivion," *Psychiatric Annals,* 3 (1973): 35.

[23] It was rumored, for example, that the lower court decision in *Bartley (Bartley v. Kremens,* 402 F.
Supp. 1039 [1975]) so threatened persons responsible for administrating inpatient psychiatric facilities
for children, that many such facilities refused to admit additional adolescent patients or even discharged
adolescent patients already admitted rather than risk the possibility of future, formal legal hearings to justify psychiatric hospitalizations of minors by their parents. Similarly, it is not clear to this author that the
patients who have been discharged from (or retained by) Bryce Hospital in Alabama in the wake of *Wyatt
(Wyatt v. Stickney,* 325 F. Supp. 781 [1971] 334 F. Supp. 781 [1971]; 344 F. Supp. 373 and 344 F.
Supp. 385 [1974]; *Wyatt v. Aderholt,* 503 F.2d 1305 [1974]) have really fared any better by virtue of
that series of class action litigations. There is even doubt that the various *Lessard* litigations in Wisconsin
(*Lessard v. Schmidt,* 349 F. Supp. 1078 [1974]; *Schmidt v. Lessard,* 414 U.S. 473 [1974]; 379 F. Supp.
1376 and 420 U.S. 592 [1975]) have resulted in visible improvements vis-a-vis civil commitment proceedings in that state.

[24] *Lynch v. Baxley,* 386 F. Supp. 378, 389 (1974).

sumption, both in America and in Poland, that many disciplines working simultaneously can analyze and resolve the complex social, legal, political and ethical problems which arise within the context of caring for mentally ill persons. All too often the magic imputed to this multidisciplinary mix is unfounded. Professionals of one discipline may not be sufficiently trained in a sister profession to communicate ideas across interdisciplinary boundaries. The confusion and misunderstanding which results in the attempt to do so often lead to unnecessary antagonisms. I suspect that the benefits to be derived from multidisciplinary endeavors on behalf of mentally ill persons cannot be fully realized at the present time. The ultimate value of such endeavors would seem instead to depend upon the degree to which various professions are willing to make systematic efforts to provide their members with interdisciplinary training and expertise. In the interim, multidisciplinary collaboration is more promise than panacea in my opinion, at least insofar as the mentally ill are concerned.

Conclusion

Despite the rather pessimistic tone of this commentary, I believe that many elements of Poland's Mental Health Draft Proposal should be viewed with optimism. There is, at the very least, the promise of more integrated and accessible mental health services for those Polish citizens who desperately require them. But at the same time the Draft Proposal may pose certain risks — to mental health professionals whose legitimate practices may be unfortunately compromised from without, to patients whose "mental disturbances" may indeed be too minor and transient to warrant the imposition of involuntary treatment, and even to the state which may ultimately fail to deliver the vast array of social benefits which it seemingly promises. But if the Draft Proposal is ultimately adopted by the Polish people, tomorrow will determine whether its risks outweigh its benefits. Therein lies the greatest challenge — to ask what impact the Draft Proposal has had following its enactment, and to share that knowledge openly with other countries. Meanwhile, Poland's Draft Proposal is undeniably a courageous step, an accomplishment in which Dr. Dabrowski, the 1974 Commission of Experts and the Polish people can take great pride.

Comments on Dabrowski's "Major Issues in the Polish Mental Health Legislation Draft Proposal"

Commentator: Larry O. Gostin*

Professor Dabrowski has taken us through a minefield of problems and difficulties in setting legislative boundaries to the provision of a mental health service in Poland. I propose to compare his solutions with those now being put forward in Great Britain.[1]

No country can shed its obligation to provide a comprehensive and humane health service for those who suffer from mental illness. Despite its humanitarian traditions, Britain now finds it is the subject of an investigation by the European Commission of Human Rights in respect of its powers of detention and of the conditions in its psychiatric institutions.[2] Other countries have faced similar international criticism.[3]

At the same time, it is improper to define social, behavioral, or political problems in psychiatric terms. The Polish Draft Proposal defines mental disorder to include "mental disease namely psychosis and mental retardation," "neurotic disturbances" and "personality disorders."[4] This appears to encompass a wide variety of people whose character, attitudes or intelligence is con-

---

*Legal Director, MIND (National Association for Mental Health), 22 Harley Street, London W1N 2ED, England.

[1] See generally, Department of Health and Social Security, *A Review of the Mental Health Act 1959* (London: HMSO, 1976).

[2] *A, B, C, and D v. United Kingdom* (Application numbers 6840/74, 6870/75, 6998/75, 7099/77). Applications A, B, and D were held admissible under articles 3 and 5 of the European Convention of Human Rights in May 1977. (The decision in application C was reserved.) An article written by the author, who represented the four patients in these cases, will be included in a forthcoming issue of the *International Journal of Law and Psychiatry*.

[3] A case against the government of the Netherlands is also pending before the European Commission of Human Rights. Application number 6301/73. See also S. Bloch and P. Reddaway, *Russia's Political Hospitals* (London: Victor Gollancz Ltd., 1977).

[4] It is worth noting that the term "mental disorder" in the Draft Proposal is defined to include several psychiatric classifications which are themselves left undefined. "Personality disorder," for example, has not been reliably and validly defined by international standards, and has been the subject of recent criticism by the World Health Organization and World Federation of Mental Health. See, World Health Organization, *Law and Mental Health: Harmonising Objectives: Guiding Principles Based on an International Survey* (Geneva: WHO, in press). See also, T. C. N. Gibbens, "Treatment of Psychopaths," *J. Ment. Sci.* 62 (1961): 181; *The Report of the Committee on Mentally Abnormal Offenders* (London: HMSO, Cmnd. 6244, 1975), pp. 77–108.

sidered abnormal;[5] the definition does not have sufficient regard to whether the deviance can reasonably be regarded as an "illness" which is susceptible to psychiatric treatment.

The definition in the Draft Proposal does not appropriately circumscribe the kinds of people who are eligible for admission to hospital. It is therefore important to closely examine the procedures for admission, both on an informal and compulsory basis.

Informal Admission

The existing mental health regulations in Poland, together with legislation in many jurisdictions in the United States and in the Commonwealth, are modeled upon the Mental Health Act 1959 of England and Wales. A principal objective of the 1959 Act was to make treatment available to the patient when it was medically prescribed.[6] Legal safeguards were not usually required because the treatment was offered, as in a general hospital, on a voluntary or contractual basis. In fact, in Britain, and in many commonwealth jurisdictions, 85% or more of all patients are admitted without formality of any kind.[7]

There is now evidence that the analogy between psychiatric and general hospital admissions is invalid. Psychiatric facilities do not only serve medical interests but also provide homes for unwanted people,[8] training centers for physically and mentally handicapped people,[9] and refuges for the elderly.[10] Although patients may not protest, it does not mean they are genuinely content to remain in hospital or that an institutional setting is the most appropriate place to meet their needs.[11]

The proposed Polish Act gives partial recognition to this problem. If an unprotesting patient is incapable of giving consent, the hospital authorities are required to refer him or her to the Guardianship Court within 48 hours of admission. The statutory criterion used is the capacity of the patient to "understand where he is or why he was brought to hospital."

The consent required in the Proposal does not meet conventional standards of informed legal consent. First, the criterion for determining the validity of consent is demonstrably under-inclusive; only a gravely disabled person would be incapable of recognizing his surroundings. The more important issue is whether prospective patients understand what they are undertaking. There is

---

[5] See also, section 4 of the Mental Health Act (England and Wales) 1959 where "mental disorder" is defined to include "mental illness, arrested or incomplete development of mind, psychopathic disorder, *and any other disorder or disability of mind*" [emphasis added].

[6] K. Jones, *A History of the Mental Health Services* (London: Routledge and Kegan Paul, 1972).

[7] W. J. Curran, "Comparative Analysis of Mental Health Legislation in Forty-Three Countries: A Discussion of Historical Trends," *International Journal of Law and Psychiatry*, 1 (1978): 79, 86–87.

[8] See, MIND, *Evidence to the Royal Commission on the National Health Service with regard to Services for Mentally Ill and Mentally Handicapped People* (London: MIND, 1977).

[9] See, Department of Health and Social Security, *Better Services for the Mentally Handicapped* (London: HMSO, 1971, Cmnd. 4683).

[10] See, Department of Health and Social Security, *Priorities for Health and Personal Social Services in England: A Consultative Document* (London: HMSO, 1976).

[11] See generally, J. Ellis, "Volunteering Children: Parental Commitment of Minors to Mental Institutions," *Calif. L. Rev.* 62 (1974): 840.

no requirement in the Proposal to inform the patient of the forms of treatment which will be offered; the probable course or duration of the treatment; the attendant loss of rights or privileges associated with informal admission; and most importantly the procedures necessary for the patient to withdraw consent to admission or treatment.

Second, the decision on whether an informal patient will receive the safeguard afforded by the Guardianship Court is within the unreviewable discretion of the hospital authorities. Thus, the hearing intended to assess the propriety of hospital care is triggered by the self-same professional who is offering that care. The practical effect is that those hospitals which provide a low standard of care may also tend to disregard the legal interests of their patients, while the opposite may result in more progressive institutions. It is precisely those patients requiring an independent assessment who may not therefore be referred to the Guardianship Court.

The research undertaken by Professor Dabrowski lends support to these first two points. The number of patients who would be referred to the Court because of their inability to consent would range from 1.6 to 4.5% of all admissions. This figure is considerably lower than those provided in other European countries.[12] In England and Wales, for example, the government itself estimates that between one-half and two-thirds of all informal patients are not mentally ill, but remain in hospital because they have no home to go to, or for other social or domiciliary reasons.[13] There is no meaningful consent in these cases because there is no realistic choice among alternatives.

Professor Dabrowski's research also shows a wide variation among hospital authorities in their referral rates to the court. These differences may not be based as much on the condition of patients as on the attitudes and training of professionals.

Even if the criteria and procedures for determining the capacity of the patient to consent were valid, there would still remain the issue of whether the consent was made without undue influence. It is experientially self-evident that some patients agree to hospital admission because of an implied or express threat of a compulsory order. This has also been empirically demonstrated in Great Britain.[14] The proposed Polish Act therefore could usefully be amended to incorporate this aspect of informed consent.

Compulsory Admission

Under the Polish Draft Proposal, a person can be compulsorily admitted to hospital on the recommendation of one medical practitioner, who need not be a qualified psychiatrist. The hospital director is required to notify the Guardianship Court within 48 hours of admission, and the Court must hear the case within 14 days.

---

[12]See e.g., Scottish Mental Welfare Commission, *No Place to Go* (Edinburgh: HMSO, 1975).

[13]*Hansard* written parliamentary answer by Dr. David Owen, then Minister of State for Health (London: HMSO, January 15, 1976).

[14]See, Ministry of Health, *Annual Report for 1966 on the State of Public Health* (London: HMSO, 1967) 160.

It is thus apparent that there may be no judicial review of the decision to detain a person until 16 days following admission. The manifest lack of safeguards available to the patient during this period (e.g., there is no application by a social worker or relative and no need for a corroborative medical opinion) is justified in the proposed legislation by the need to act expediently in cases of emergency. But, unlike the existing regulations in Poland, there is no element of "urgent necessity" within the proposed legislation, and one is left with the impression that the simplicity of procedure is intended more as a measure of administrative convenience. Further, genuine emergencies do not normally extend for a period of 16 days. Even if in the rare case this were true (as in a severe endogenous depression, not immediately responding to medical intervention), it would still not justify the inadequacy of protection afforded the great majority of patients. Detention without legal recourse for a period exceeding two weeks will no doubt be seen by the patient as an affront to his or her liberty and dignity.

Empirical studies in the United Kingdom suggest that similar emergency provisions[15] (although they expire within 72 hours unless a second medical opinion is obtained) are subject to misuse.[16] General practitioners, who usually operate emergency procedures, have been shown to have particular difficulty in assessing the psychiatric element in a person's medical or social condition, especially when called on at night or in an emergency.[17]

More recent studies show that between 60% and 80% of all such admissions are considered unjustified by psychiatric and social work assessors.[18] This points to the minimal need for a corroborative professional opinion, which can reasonably be expected within 24 hours following an emergency admission.

A more interesting phenomenon in Britain is that professionals are shaping the duration of confinement to periods of time which will not require them to justify their decisions to legal authorities.[19] In 1975, 97% of the people compulsorily admitted to hospital were ineligible for Mental Health Review Tribunals, because they were discharged within the 28-day limit provided under the 1959 Act.[20] It is conceivable, therefore, that the 16-day period in the Draft proposal will itself take on an artificial significance in Polish psychiatry. The patient, of course, will suffer because the psychiatrist's discharge decision may be influenced by a desire to circumvent the intended legal safeguards, rather than by a clinical assessment of the patient's response to treatment.

---

[15] Mental Health Act (England and Wales) 1959, s. 29.

[16] See e.g., R. Barton and J. Haider, "Unnecessary Compulsory Admission to a Psychiatric Hospital," *Med. Sci. Law* 6 (1966): 147.

[17] M. Clybe, *Night Calls* (London: 1962).

[18] P. Bean, "Are Mental Health Guardians Abusing their Power?" *The Times* (London) (January 3, 1978).

[19] L. O. Gostin, *The Mental Health Act 1959: Is it Fair?* (London: MIND, 1978).

[20] Mental Health Review Tribunals are independent administrative authorities, comprised of a legal chairman and a medical and a lay member, which are empowered to discharge patients detained, *inter alia* under section 26 of the Mental Health Act 1959. Section 26 authorizes admission for one year, and may be renewed by the responsible medical officer for one further year and, thereafter, for two years at a time. Patients detained under short term orders for 72 hours (sections 29, 30, 135 and 136) or under a medium term order for 28 days (section 25) are not eligible to apply for tribunals. For the most recent statistical breakdown of the use of these sections see, Department of Health and Social Security, *Inpatient Statistics from the Mental Health Enquiry for England, 1975* (London: HMSO, 1978).

In Britain, of those few patients who have recourse to Mental Health Review Tribunals only about 12% actually apply for a hearing. There are many reasons for this ranging from their misunderstanding of the procedure, to their confusion, vulnerability and apathy.[21] The European Commission of Human Rights, in *obiter dicta* in the United Kingdom cases, suggested that review procedures should not rely on the initiative of patients, but should occur *ex officio.*[22]

The access to review procedures under the Draft Proposal of Poland is comparable to those under the British Act. Under the Draft Proposal, the initial determination of the Guardianship Court is made *ex officio.* Thereafter, there is no time limit within which the powers of detention automatically cease and procedures for renewal are operated. Rather, the patient is detained indefinitely and the burden of applying for subsequent hearings shifts from the State to the patient. As the British experience demonstrates, patients will seldom take the initiative to exercise their right to a hearing.

Conclusion

The Draft Proposal of Poland ostensibly attempts a resolution of problems relating to hospital admission which have plagued a variety of jurisdictions in Europe and North America. It does not ignore the issue of consent to informal admission as in most countries, but the proposed standard is unlikely to protect the uninformed and vulnerable patient who resides in a hospital but does not benefit from a medical environment. So too, the Guardianship Court has all the trappings of an effective safeguard of the liberty of the subject. But the safeguard may not operate until the patient has been forcibly detained and treated for 16 days; thereafter it will only operate at the initiative of the patient who has shown a reluctance to exercise his rights in other jurisdictions.

---

[21] For a complete analysis and discussion of the figures pertaining to tribunal application rates in England and Wales, see L. O. Gostin, *A Human Condition: The Mental Health Act from 1959 to 1975, Observations, Analysis and Proposals for Reform,* vol. 1 (London: MIND, 1975). It is also of interest to examine the practices of other countries which have adopted the 1959 Act, either in full or in part. In some of these countries, although many thousands of patients are eligible to apply for tribunals, only a handful actually exercise the right. In one country, Mauritius, there has never been a tribunal hearing.

[22] *A, B, C, and D v. United Kingdom, supra,* note 2.

The Politics of Mental Health Advocacy in the United States

Patricia M. Wald* and Paul R. Friedman**

During the 1970s in the United States we have seen a dramatic confrontation between the mental health and the legal system. Litigation brought by advocates on behalf of mentally ill and mentally retarded persons has sparked what is often referred to as a revolutionary "patients' rights" movement. In half a decade, mentally handicapped persons have been successful in persuading federal courts that they have a right to treatment,[1] to protection from harm,[2] to treatment in the "least restrictive setting,"[3] to equal educational opportunity,[4] to protection from forced administration of hazardous or intrusive procedures,[5] to both procedural and substantive protections in the civil commitment process,[6] to safeguards against indefinite confinement after a finding that they are incompetent to stand trial,[7] and to liberty.[8] The essence of these landmark judicial decisions has been incorporated into both state laws and federal legislation such as the Education of All Handicapped Children Act of 1975,[9] the Rehabilitation Act of 1973,[10] and the Developmentally Disabled Bill of Rights and Assistance Act of 1975.[11]

---

*Assistant Attorney General for Legislative Affairs in the United States Department of Justice, Washington, D.C.

**Managing Attorney and President of the Mental Health Law Project, Washington, D.C. The views expressed in this paper are the personal views of the authors and do not reflect any official policy of the Justice Department or the Mental Health Law Project.

[1] e.g., *Rouse v. Cameron*, 387 F.2d 241 (D.C. Cir. 1967); *Wyatt v. Stickney*, 325 F. Supp. 781, 784 (M.D. Ala. 1971), 334 F. Supp. 1341 (M.D. Ala. 1971), 344 F. Supp. 373 and 387 (M.D. Ala. 1972), aff'd *sub nom Wyatt v. Aderholt*, 503 F.2d 1305 (5th Cir. 1974); *Welsch v. Likins*, 373 F. Supp. 487, 493 (D. Minn. 1974), further proceedings at 550 F.2d 1122 (8th Cir. 1977); *Davis v. Watkins*, 384 F. Supp. 1196, 1203–1212 (N.D. Ohio 1974).

[2] e.g., *New York State Association for Retarded Children, Inc. v. Rockefeller*, 357 F. Supp. 752, 764 (E.D.N.Y. 1973), consent judgment approved *sub nom New York State Association for Retarded Children, Inc. v. Carey*, 393 F. Supp. 715 (E.D. N.Y. 1975) [hereafter the "NYSARC" or "Willowbrook" case.]

[3] e.g., *Dixon v. Weinberger*, 405 F. Supp. 974 (D.D.C. 1975).

[4] e.g., *Pennsylvania Association for Retarded Children v. Pennsylvania*, 334 F. Supp. 1257 (E.D. Pa. 1971); *Mills v. Board of Education*, 348 F. Supp. 866 (D.D.C. 1972).

[5] e.g., *Kaimowitz v. Michigan Department of Mental Health*, Civil No. 73-19434-AW, 42 U.S.L.W. 2063 (Mich. Cir. Ct. 1973); *Scott v. Plante*, 532 F. 2d 939, 946 (3d Cir. 1976).

[6] e.g., *Lessard v. Schmidt*, 349 F. Supp. 1078 (E.D. Wisc. 1972) [subsequent history omitted]; *Lynch v. Baxley* 386 F. Supp. 378 (M.D. Ala. 1974) (3 Judge Court); *Bell v. Wayne County General Hospital*, 384 F. Supp. 1085 (E.D. Mich. 1974) (3 Judge Court).

[7] *Jackson v. Indiana*, 406 U.S. 715 (1972).

[8] *O'Connor v. Donaldson*, 422 U.S. 563 (1975).

[9] P.L. 94-142, 10 U.S.C. sec. 1401 *et seq.* (1975).

[10] 29 U.S.C. sec. 701 *et seq.*, as amended (Supp. IV, 1974); regulations codified at 45 CFR Part 84 (1977).

[11] 42 U.S.C. sec. 6010 *et. seq.* (1975).

From a distance these developments may look like steady and inexorable progress. But along both sides of the apparently smooth surface of this path lurks a tangle of tensions between competing values, between various professions and among the branches of government which make up the American political machine. The advocacy movement has created a disequilibrium in a complex force field, and it is still too early to know what the mental health system will look like when and if a balance is once again established. In this article we will briefly explore three of the major tensions which have characterized a half decade of breakthrough developments in mental health law in the United States.

A. The Courts versus the Executive and Legislative Branches of Government as Agent for Reform

Before exploring the tensions created by efforts at judicial rather than legislative or executive reform, it is necessary to look back for a moment at how our courts have become so embroiled with the mental health system.

Until the late 1960s, law and psychiatry intersected primarily around issues of criminal behavior and forensics. The critical focus was on what to do about a specialized kind of offender within the bounds of the familiar criminal law system.[12] Only a few voices railed about what was happening to those troubled souls in our mental hospitals who were not alleged to have committed offenses.[13] A few intrepid watchers recoiled at Frederick Weisman's documentary film, "Titticut Follies," and investigative journalists would periodically discover a "Willowbrook." But we resolutely used the defenses of avoidance and denial to convince ourselves that the snakepit was actually a rosegarden in which a magical visiting psychiatrist would save the chronic, backward schizophrenics. In short, the American perception was still one of psychiatric omniscience and wondrous psychotropics.

There were, of course, pioneers such as Senator Ervin of North Carolina, whose District of Columbia Hospitalization of the Mentally Ill Act in 1964[14] provided a court hearing and a right to counsel for anyone subject to commitment for mental illness, legislated certain patient rights and even included a little-understood but long-remembered phrase about a "right to treatment."[15] But on the whole, courts and lawyers ventured only occasionally into the civil mental health system.

In 1973, the Supreme Court recognized what had been a long-standing injustice: the indefinite confinement of persons held "incompetent to stand trial"

---

[12]e.g., A. Goldstein, *The Insanity Defense* (1967); Burt and Morris, "A Proposal for the Abolition of the Incompetency Plea," *Univ. Chicago Law Review* 40 (1972): 66.

[13]e.g., A. Deutsch, *The Mentally Ill in America*, 2nd ed. (1949); T. Szasz, *Law, Liberty and Psychiatry* (1963); D. Rothman, *Discovery of the Asylum* (1971).

[14]D.C. Code sec. 21-501 to 21-509 (Supp. IV 1966).

[15]See Birnbaum, "The Right to Treatment," *Amer. Bar Assn. Journal* 46 (1960): 499. The first major case dealing with a patient's rights within the mental hospital concerned one Charles Rouse who had entered St. Elizabeth's Hospital on a "not guilty by reason of insanity" committal. In 1967, he sued for release because he was not receiving any treatment and the Court declared he had an enforceable right to "suitable treatment . . . adequate in light of present knowledge" under the 1964 D.C. Act and perhaps under the Constitution of the United States. *Rouse v. Cameron,* 373 F.2d 451, 456 (D.C. Cir. 1967).

for reasons of retardation or mental illness without options for either trial on the merits or a regular civil commitment process.[16] After briefly discussing the wide variation in state commitment statutes, the Supreme Court commented prophetically that "considering the number of persons affected, it is perhaps remarkable that the substantive constitutional limitations on this [commitment] power have not been more frequently litigated."[17]

During this period in the United States, we witnessed both rapid expansion of legal services for the poor and a federal program to repay defenders of the criminally accused in federal courts.[18] The advances earned by poverty lawyers in the courts – acknowledged to be the most successful part of our much-vaunted "War on Poverty" – were eyed enviously by the advocates of other disadvantaged groups, often frustrated by lack of results from "team-playing" with local mental health officials and the professionals. The poverty lawyers themselves encountered numerous cases of clients embroiled in the mental health system, resisting commitment, alleging discrimination in the community or complaining of institutional brutality or neglect.

In these years, the patient, parent and relative organizations representing the mentally ill and retarded formed a loose alliance with the lawyer-advocates. They became a stable source of clients for test cases involving the rights of the mentally handicapped.

The stage for these actions was set by several decades of growing disenchantment with the therapeutic benefits of large impersonal mental health hospitals, typically located in rural surroundings far away from patients' families, from employment and even from access to skilled personnel. Abuses of patients in such institutions often flourished because of their isolation. The advent of the psychotropics in the 1950s resulted in a major reduction of the institutional population. But many patients like Kenneth Donaldson – the plaintiff in the landmark 1973 Supreme Court case cited above – were incontestably maintained in incarceration for needless and heartbreaking years because they had provoked the ire of their caretakers or because there were not resources to treat them outside. Countless studies documented that our state mental hospitals were a national scandal.[19]

In 1971, a courageous federal judge took a radical step. After personally touring a very substandard institution in Alabama – and after listening to a parade of experts declare what minimum environmental and personal resources were necessary for even the possibility of treatment – Judge Frank Johnson declared the entire hospital setting to be an unconstitutional deprivation of the rights of patients to be "treated."[20] The basic idea was that, under the due pro-

---

[16] *Jackson v. Indiana*, 406 U.S. 715 (1972).

[17] *Id.* at 737.

[18] Criminal Justice Act, 18 U.S.C. sec. 3006A (1970).

[19] See, e.g., *NYSARC, supra* note 2, at 756; *Wyatt, supra* note 1, 344 F. Supp. at 391 and 394. Peskze, *Involuntary Treatment of the Mentally Ill* (1975): 67. A. A. Stone, *Mental Health and Law: A System in Transition* (NIMH 1975): 88, 121. National Assn. of Superintendents, *Current Trends and Status of Public Residential Services for the Mentally Retarded* (1975); Advisory Committee on Child Development of the National Science Foundation, *Toward a National Policy for Children and Families* (1976): 117–119.

[20] *Wyatt, supra* note 1, 325 F. Supp. 781 (M.D. Ala. 1971).

cess clause, adequate and effective treatment was the *quid pro quo* for their involuntary commitment. The lawsuits against understaffed, underfinanced, inhumane state facilities (for both the mentally ill and the mentally retarded) multiplied. Federal district judges laid down long lists of specific standards with which state institutions must comply if they were to stay in business.

A recent extension of such suits has been the demand that states not only maintain desirable conditions and levels of skilled personnel in state institutions but that they create or finance alternatives to those institutions as well. The theory for such suits is found in the Fifth Amendment guarantee of due process, which means (as judicially interpreted) that even if the state's purpose for restricting an individual's liberty is a legitimate one, it must be accomplished in the least restrictive way possible. Therefore, persons deprived of liberty for the sake of treatment must be treated in the least restrictive setting that is suitable to their condition – and states cannot limit their treatment facilities to massive institutions when community-based treatment would do the job as well.

While treatment cases were going on, other class-action test cases were establishing that exclusion of mentally retarded children from state school systems violated their constitutional rights under the equal protection clause, and courts were requiring defendants to make extensive outreach efforts to identify and place previously excluded children and to provide them with an education suitable to their individual needs.

The *Wyatt* case provides a good illustration of tensions between judicial and legislative or executive reform. On the appeal of the *Wyatt* decision to the Fifth Circuit, the State of Alabama took the position that the kind of decree rendered by Judge Johnson constituted an illegal infringement upon the functions of the State legislature. The governor and the legislature were upset first by the high cost of implementing minimum standards and, secondly, by the alleged usurpation of a legislative function – the balancing of the needs of mental patients against other equally important demands upon State revenues, such as old-age pensions, welfare payments and renovated highways. To the plaintiffs, the question was whether constitutional rights were to be vindicated. Many constitutionally based decisions require reallocation of financial resources. Lack of adequate financial resources has never been accepted as a valid justification for the denial of a constitutional right. The cases have made clear that whether a state decides to run a mental health system is entirely within its own discretion, but once it decides to undertake this function, it must do so in a manner which does not violate constitutional rights.

As both defendants and plaintiffs recognized, the critical issue underlying class-action right-to-treatment or right-to-education cases is one of judicial control of financing. The effort by patient advocates is to force the legislatures to reallocate their fiscal priorities. When the State of Alabama contended that it simply lacked the funds to finance the physical-plant improvements and increased staffing ratios ordered by Judge Johnson, George Dean, the wily lawyer for the plaintiffs, did some hurried research. He discovered that for the current fiscal year, the State of Alabama had already appropriated substantial sums for such diverse activities as a White House of the Confederacy, an Alabama Junior Miss Pageant, a livestock coliseum, and a Sports Hall of Fame. Then, to dramatize the issue of fiscal priorities, he typed up a bristling pleading which he filed with the Court and made available to the press, contending that his clients would be better treated in Alabama if they were "athletic or photogenic cows of Confederate ancestry."[21]

Most of the judges in the first wave of reform cases consciously deferred decision on the ultimate question of what they would do if the state legislatures refused to vote the money necessary to meet the new standards. Cries of "judicial usurpation" and "federal tyranny" mounted, however, as such constitutional confrontations came nearer. Can a federal court really order a state government to allocate a specified amount of money to its mental health system at the expense of its schools, highways, public health or other social welfare systems? What can the federal court do if the state simply refuses? Can it hold state legislators in contempt — or, if not a legislator, then at least the state treasurer — for failure to disburse necessary funds? We still do not know the answer; the poker game is still going on. At stake are some very basic notions about the proper role of the judiciary vis-a-vis the legislature and of the federal government versus the states in a system based upon the cardinal principle of separation of powers and a form of federalism in which the central government is to exercise powers expressly conferred on it by the states.[22]

The underlying issue of fiscal control has in turn led critics of the new judicial activism in mental health to question the real motivation for such lawsuits. Are they what they seem to be: attempts to humanize a traumatic experience for patients and assure them whatever chance for recovery the state of the art permits? Or are they — as many allege — a stratagem to bring institutional operations to a halt so that involuntary commitment will cease? Or to embarrass a particular political figure such as the governor? Or, more moderately, do such lawsuits simply attempt to insist that the full costs of decent hospitalization be weighed fairly against the allegedly lower costs of community care? The motivation undoubtedly varies with the lawyer and the clients, but the overriding result of such suits is that the courts in America — particularly the federal courts — have become power brokers invading the formerly "political" territory of state governors and legislatures and deciding how state resources will be allocated both within the mental health system and between that and other state systems.

On balance, then, is there a sufficient justification for this legal incursion into areas that are traditionally ones of executive and legislative discretion? There is no pat answer except the historical imperative. In the past decade the courts in America have become the last and often the best bastion of the defenseless. That status could be changing today under a heavy assault from constitutional conservatives who deplore such activism from the "least powerful branch." The mentally ill have not traditionally been very successful in displaying clout with politicians or legislatures; their advances have been grounded in

---

[21] See plaintiff's "Motion to Add Persons Needed for Just Adjudication," filed with the United States District Court on September 1, 1971.

[22] See, e.g., the opinion of the 8th Circuit in the appeal of *Welsch v. Likins, supra* note 1, 550 F.2d 1122 (1977).

basic principles of fairness and equity, traditionally the province of the courts. If the power of courts to influence the mental health systems is cut back, they will almost surely suffer.

It is, additionally, a time-honored function of courts to supervise trustees and guardians and hold them accountable; in a modern urban society, courts may have to assume the same supervisory duties over state custodians of the mentally ill. What they need to do is to find more efficient ways to perform those duties — perhaps a corps of court-employed inspectors or masters.

The success of attempts to use judicial power to change the system will continue to depend on the availability of lawyers to represent such clients and such causes and upon the receptivity of a federal judiciary to approve such challenges.

The situation is decidedly fluid. Congress has before it legislation to increase dramatically the number of federal judges,[23] to be appointed by a President whose wife heads a special "President's Commission on Mental Health." It is also considering legislation which would allow attorney's fees to be granted in successful lawsuits brought by mental health advocates in the public interest.[24] Another bill currently pending before the Congress would authorize the Department of Justice to bring suits in federal courts to protect the rights of mental patients.[25] It is vehemently opposed by the state attorneys general, purportedly because of their concern for preserving our federalistic system. If enacted, it will permit the resources of the federal government, including the Federal Bureau of Investigation, to be brought ot bear against institutional deprivation of constitutional rights. The level of funding and the priorities of the Legal Services Corporation also will influence the development of mental health law.[26]

While the scope of advocacy efforts is this uncertain, we do not expect to see a cessation of attempts to use judicial power to change the system.

B. Tensions within the Legal Advocacy System: The Service-Oriented versus the Civil Rights Perspective

Increasingly in the United States the mentally ill, the mentally retarded and the physically handicapped perceive themselves — and are politically perceived — as a minority group who have been historically denied basic civil liberties such as the right to liberty and the rights to vote, to marry, to bear children, to be employed, to go to school. Their campaigns resemble in method and legal theory those of other disadvantaged groups — racial, religious and sexual — in American politics. For their court victories, they have relied upon the same clauses of the United States Constitution, those requiring due process before liberty may be infringed and those mandating equal protection of the laws. The organized groups in the forefront of mental health law reform include the Civil Liberties Union and the Mental Health Law Project. The Civil Rights Division of the United States Department of Justice, which enforces constitutional and

---

[23] The Judgeships Bill, HR 7843, passed by the House of Representatives, February 7, 1978.

[24] See, e.g., The Federal Court Attorney's Fees Act of 1977, HR 10105, 95th Congress, 1st Session.

[25] HR 9400, now pending before the Judiciary Committee of the House of Representatives. The parallel bill in the Senate is S 1393.

[26] Legal Services Act of 1974, 42 U.S.C. sec. 2996-2996 (L), amended by Pub. Laws 93-355 and 95-222, Dec. 28, 1977.

statutory nondiscrimination rights of racial and sexual groups, has a special section to ensure the rights of persons in mental institutions and in prisons and jails.

At the same time, however, mentally handicapped persons in the United States have increasingly come to view themselves as part of another movement of equally profound consequence for Americans: the consumer movement. Perhaps best typified by the figure of Ralph Nader — with his campaign to ensure the safety of automobiles, the purity of food products and the truth of advertisements — the consumer movement aims generally to improve the quality and quantity of services which large corporations and government are charged with delivering to citizens. Like environmentalists, shoppers and welfare recipients, mentally handicapped persons with their friends and advocates have organized into interest groups such as the Mental Health Association, the National Association for Retarded Citizens and a number of local ex-patient groups to demand that the state provide more and better mental health services.

On the surface, one would not expect the civil rights and consumerism approaches to mental health advocacy to create many difficulties or inconsistencies. And indeed in many instances they have reinforced each other. But at times the two currents do push in opposing directions, setting up acute tensions within the advocacy network. Consider, for example, the conflicting attitudes of civil libertarians and service-oriented advocates concerning the proper use of civil commitment to compel involuntary treatment of the mentally ill.

Civil commitment is grounded on two doctrinal bases: police power and parental (*parens patriae*) power. The police power rests upon the need to protect society from the acts of dangerous mentally handicapped persons. Parental power (*parens patriae*) rests upon the need of the mentally handicapped for help and treatment.[27] Most states require for commitment that a person be either mentally ill and dangerous to himself or others, or mentally ill and in need of treatment. Not surprisingly, given their different philosophical orientations, civil libertarian and services-oriented advocates take radically different positions with regard to the legitimacy of these two traditional justifications for civil commitment.

Civil libertarians note that whatever the alleged benefits of mental health interventions through civil commitment, there is major potential for harm as well. The most obvious harm stemming from civil commitment is its "massive curtailment of liberty."[28] The loss of physical freedom resulting from civil commitment is, for all practical purposes, little different from that which results from a prison sentence. Depending upon the quality of the hospital, a person committed may be subject to overcrowding, unsanitary conditions, poor nutrition and even to brutality at the hands of attendants or other hospital residents. Commitment also infringes grossly upon privacy, and committed patients may be subjected to compulsory medication, electroconvulsive therapy and other potentially hazardous and intrusive procedures. Furthermore, hospitalization is disruptive of family, social and economic ties and ex-mental patients,

---

[27]See generally "Developments in the Law — Civil Commitment of the Mentally Ill," *Harvard Law Review* 87 (9174): 1193, 1201-1245.

[28]*Humphrey v. Cady*, 405 U.S. 504, 509 (1972).

like ex-convicts, can expect routinely to encounter severe stigma and active discrimination when they return to the community.

For civil libertarians, then, the notion that the state may deprive someone of liberty for his or her own good is to be treated with extreme suspicion. As a highly respected Justice of the United States Supreme Court has written, "[e]xperience should teach us to be most on our guard to protect liberty when the government's purposes are beneficient . . . [t]he greatest dangers to liberty lurk in insidious encroachment by men of zeal, well-meaning, but without understanding."[29]

The civil libertarians would abolish civil commitment based upon paternalism alone because they fear its application is overbroad and often based on circular reasoning. ("Mr. X is mentally ill and incompetent to make treatment decisions because he disputes the doctor's diagnosis and recommendation.") The right to eat garbage, to exist in perpetual anxiety, to live in the gutters or bus stations or be a "shopping bag lady" wandering aimlessly from hallway to alley, often the prey of street predators — they argue — is still a valuable right. The right to be deviant and eccentric, even to deny oneself valuable services, must be staunchly defended, or else there is a danger that the civil commitment system will be used to enforce the values, lifestyles or ideologies of the powerful and the majority against the powerless and the minority.[30] This apprehension about the logical extremes of the *parens patriae* rationale is not without some basis, as evidenced by the contemporary corruption of mental health systems in totalitarian countries, where they have become alternative Siberias or Gulag Archipelagoes for political dissenters. While mental institutions in the United States do not appear to be systematically used in this way, there is enough evidence of similar abuses in individual cases to justify concern.

Civil libertarians conclude that unless a person is physically dangerous, the state has no legitimate purpose in confining him and imposing treatment against his will. A few federal courts have accepted this constitutional attack on the *parens patriae* power, thus effectively limiting civil commitment to those who are dangerous.[31] Several states have also amended their statutes to conform with this position.[32]

But the civil libertarians have problems with the police power justification for civil commitment as well. In their view, this rationale is undercut by the inability of mental health professionals accurately to predict dangerousness and by their well-documented tendency to err on the side of overprediction.[33] Fur-

---

[29] Justice Brandeis, in dissent, *Olmstead v. United States,* 277 U.S. 438, 479 (1928).

[30] See, e.g., *O'Connor v. Donaldson, supra* note 8 at 575. "May the State fence in the harmless mentally ill solely to save its citizens from exposure to those whose ways are different? One might as well ask if the State, to avoid public unease, could incarcerate all who are physically unattractive or socially eccentric. Mere public intolerance or animosity cannot constitutionally justify the deprivation of a person's physical liberty."

[31] See cases cited *supra* note 6.

[32] e.g., Cal. Welf: and Institution's Code sec. 5300 *et seq.* Deering 1969; Rev. Code of Washington sec. 71.05.280 *et seq.* (1974). For a survey of State laws, see "Developments," *supra,* note 1, at 1203–1204.

[33] See e.g., Ennis and Litwack, "Psychiatry and the Presumption of Expertise: Flipping Coins in the Courtroom," *California Law Review* 62 (1974): 693; American Psychiatric Assn., "Task Force Report No. 8: Clinical Aspects of the Violent Individual," (1975). Hunt and Wiley, "Operation Baxtrom after

thermore, they feel that, even in jurisdictions which technically authorize commitment only upon a finding of serious dangerousness, courts can and do distort the "dangerousness" criterion so as to justify commitment under a covert standard of "in need of treatment."

Services-oriented mental health advocates take a different approach to civil commitment, which more closely approximates that of mental health professionals. What the mental health system does best, they say, is to treat the treatable − not to guard the dangerous who may not be treatable. Sometimes a short period of treatment can restore agonized individuals to a productive life; why should that second chance be denied them because they are so sick they do not know enough to seek it voluntarily? Later on, they will be grateful.[34] Therefore the grounds for involuntary confinement or treatment should be probability of help, not danger to society. These spokesmen agree that the mental health system has become the unwilling repository for the old and the sick and for infirm persons who cannot cope with the demands of life and who generally need social and human services more than mental health treatment. But, they argue, in the acknowledged absence of adequate social services, we are not doing such persons any favor when we dump them onto the streets with no help or protection from the terrors and indignities of urban life. They are only left to "die with their rights on."[35]

Services-oriented advocates note that at present there is no enforceable constitutional or statutory right to adequate and effective mental health care on a voluntary basis for all citizens in our country; under the substantive due process theory − in which the right to treatment is the *quid pro quo* for the deprivation of liberty − it is only those who are involuntarily deprived of liberty by the state who have a clearly established right to treatment. Thus their involuntary confinement is the *sine qua non* to getting courts to recognize the right to better treatment inside hospitals and even after release into the community. Furthermore, the morale in a mental health system geared to treating the treatable will be far superior to that in one geared only to warehousing the dangerous.

This choice between total abolition or a "dangerousness only" standard for civil commitment on the one hand and an "in need of treatment" standard on the other will obviously have profound consequences for mental patients and for the contours of the mental health system. If a dangerousness standard is accepted and commitment is limited to cases involving imminent danger of serious bodily harm to self or others, based upon a recent overt act, society would have no authority for intervening in the lives of most current mental patients.

One Year," *Amer. Journal of Psychiatry* 124 (1968): 974; Steadman and Keveles, "The Community Adjustment and Crucial Activity of the Baxtrom Patients: 1966−1970," *Amer. Journal of Psychiatry* 129 (1972): 304; Diamond, "Dangerousness," *Univ. Pa. Law Review* 123 (1975): 439; Dershowitz, "The Psychiatrist's Power in Civil Commitment: A Knife that Cuts Both Ways," *Psychology Today* 2 (Feb. 1969): 43.

[34] For a well articulated version of the "Thank you Theory of Civil Commitment," see Alan Stone, *supra* note 20 at 70.

[35] Treffert, "Dying with their Rights On," *Prism* (1974): 47; Rachlin, "One Right Too Many," *Bulletin American Academy Psychiatry and Law* 3 (1975): 95.

From a civil libertarian viewpoint, this is a result devoutly to be sought.[36]

These two viewpoints clashed most notably in strategy sessions preceding the landmark litigation in *Wyatt v. Stickney*.[37] The conditions at Bryce Hospital in Alabama were horrible, albeit not atypical of those in other institutions around the United States. At the time of the litigation, there were three part-time psychiatrists, two social workers and one Ph.D. psychologist for 5,000 patients, an average expenditure of 50¢ per day per patient for food and a physical environment easily classified as dangerous. Services-oriented advocates felt that immediate action was necessary to establish a constitutional right to treatment and to set minimum physical-plant, nutritional and other standards to prevent physical harm to residents as well as to provide adequate and effective therapy and rehabilitation services. More civil libertarian-oriented advocates, while aware of the desperate plight of Bryce's residents, expressed great concern that right to treatment litigation would indirectly have the effect of legitimating institutions in general and thereby propping up the civil commitment process. A compromise allowed the litigation to go forward: The civil libertarians, aware that as a practical matter the people of the United States were not ready to abandon the civil commitment process, decided that forcing states to provide substantially more physical resources to institutionalized persons could be justified as creating a disincentive to unnecessary institutionalization and would cut down on the overuse of commitment, albeit not eliminating it.

There has also been contention between civil-libertarian and services-oriented advocates around efforts to establish that mental patients have a right to be treated in the least restrictive setting necessary to accomplish legitimate state goals. On its face, the notion is hard to quarrel with. The principle of the least restrictive alternative might require a daily visit by a social worker to a disturbed recluse, a hot meal or clean-linen service for those who neglect themselves, community guardianship services for those who cannot or will not bank checks, shop and pay for groceries, or community-based care homes for those who tend to wander the streets at night or forget to take necessary medicine. But again, civil libertarians fear that the obvious benefits of these services may be outweighed by the risk of ever-expanding state control over citizens' lives. Because the deprivation of liberty is less in community-based treatment than in total institutionalization — they say — the resistance against state intrusion will also be less and the lives of many more persons may ultimately be interfered with by the state, even if to a lesser extent. As a result, civil liberty-oriented advocates would eschew such suits while services-oriented advocates see them as valuable leverage in securing a diversified range of community-based services for the mentally handicapped as alternatives to institutionalization.[38]

Despite these examples, civil libertarians and services-oriented advocates

---

[36]For an excellent summary of the civil liberties and services-oriented advocacy perspectives for reform of civil commitment, compare Klein, "Mental Health Law: Legal Doctrine at the Crossroads," *Mental Health Law Project Summary of Activities* (March 1976): 7–10 with Scott, "Another Look at the Crossroads," *Mental Health Law Project Summary of Activities* (June 1976): 7–10.

[37]*Supra,* note 1, 325 F. Supp. at 783 and 334 F. Supp. at 1343.

[38]See, e.g., the statement of differing advocacy perspectives in Ewing and Hansen, "Viewpoint: The Least Restrictive Alternative," *Mental Health Law Project Summary of Activities* (Summer 1977).

have in fact worked very well together in spearheading a wide variety of mental health reforms. For example, while they may differ on the advisability of a "dangerousness" versus an "in need of treatment" standard for civil commitment, both civil libertarian and consumer-oriented advocates agree that commitment should only be authorized if a full panoply of due process procedures are employed. Test case litigation by these advocates has established, with some variation from case to case, that procedural protections must include a prompt commitment hearing preceded by adequate notice to interested parties, the right to retained or (for indigents) assigned counsel, the right to a retained or assigned independent evaluator, a transcript of the proceedings, application of the principle of the least restrictive alternative, a relatively stringent standard of proof (at least clear and convincing evidence) and the right to an expedited appeal.[39]

Both the civil liberties and consumer approaches to mental health reform also have concerns which go beyond the conditions under which the mentally ill person's liberty can be taken away. Both kinds of advocates agree that the mentally or physically handicapped child has as much right as any other child to publicly supported services such as schooling, federal or state employment eligibility, public housing and training programs. They also agree that the state must provide the special services that will make the schooling, employment or training "suitable" for the handicapped person. On this theory, a virtual educational revolution has been built in the states to guarantee mentally and physically handicapped children a right to schooling.

In *Mills v. Board of Education*,[40] one of the landmark right-to-education cases, for example, the plaintiffs were school-age children who resided in the District of Columbia and had been denied placement in publicly supported educational programs for substantial periods because of alleged physical or mental handicaps. Plaintiffs claimed that their exclusion denied them equal protection under the United States Constitution and violated statutes and regulations of the District of Columbia's Code. The court agreed and ordered the District of Columbia to make outreach efforts to identify handicapped children, take appropriate action to place such children — "mainstreaming" them where possible — and establish due process safeguards for the placement of children in special classes or programs.

Subsequently, the Education of All Handicapped Children Act of 1975 has required all states receiving federal school aid to provide an appropriate education for all the handicapped children in the state.[41] The law applies both to the handicapped children who are out of school and not receiving educational services and to handicapped children who are enrolled in school but who are not receiving programs and services adequate to meet their needs. Under this law, states are required to develop plans with the following components: Provision of "full educational opportunities" to all; due process safeguards which aid parents in challenging decisions regarding the education of their children; a guarantee that handicapped children will be educated in the "mainstream" to the fullest possible extent; procedures to assure that tests and other materials

---

[39] See note 6, *supra*.
[40] *Supra*, note 4.
[41] See notes 9, 10 *supra*.

used to evaluate a child's special needs are not culturally or racially biased; and a plan to identify and evaluate all children in the state who have special needs.

In these efforts, as well as in efforts to prohibit employment discrimination, housing discrimination and other forms of discrimination and to uphold voting rights, licensing eligibility, etc., the tension between the civil-liberties and service viewpoints has been minimal or nonexistent. Nonetheless, as the efforts of reformers attack "second wave" problems in mental health reform more subtle than the gross injustices and outrages of substandard institutions and total lack of community-based services, the differences in approach may become more important and may increasingly disrupt coalitions of rights-minded and services-oriented advocates.

C. Lawyers versus Mental Health Professionals:
   Is the Patient the Victim of Internecine Warfare Between Professionals?

While legal advocates for mentally handicapped persons have often worked closely and successfully with leading mental health professionals in planning test-case litigation, colleagues of these professionals — in some cases, the very same professionals — have eventually become the object of the lawsuits. Two controversial foci of recent legal attacks have been mental health professionals' claimed expertise in certain areas and the conflicting roles which mental health professionals discharge under our present system.

The first focus is illustrated by cases challenging the psychiatric expertise in predicting dangerousness. Traditionally, where civil commitment statutes require a finding that a person is mentally ill and dangerous, psychiatrists have been given free rein as expert witnesses to testify in court on the likelihood that a particular individual will commit a dangerous act in the future. Recently, however, legal advocates have marshaled research literature to show that there is at present no knowledge or technique which makes possible the consistently accurate prediction of future dangerous behavior and that, in comparative studies involving other professionals and even lay persons, psychiatrists are no more successful at making such predictions.[42] While some distinguished psychiatric spokesmen have in fact recognized this limitation and have expressed relief at the prospect of ceasing to function as experts in this capacity, many others have reacted with anger and defensiveness. Perhaps they feel that any loss of power in this limited respect would diminish their status and prestige generally.

At stake is much more than the right to speak as an expert on the limited issue of dangerousness. Psychiatrists have traditionally stood at the apex of the mental health profession's pyramid and clinical psychologists or social workers wishing, for example, to receive health insurance reimbursement for providing services have often had to work under the supervision of an M.D. But now the other mental health professionals are beginning to challenge the preeminence of the psychiatrists on a variety of fronts. In the civil commitment context, the medical model itself has come under a withering attack by proponents of a more behaviorally oriented model of mental illness which would condition commitment on clearly specified acts rather than on vague diagnostic criteria.

---

[42] See note 33, *supra*.

Legal advocates are not only scrutinizing allegedly exaggerated claims of expertise but are also showing an increasing concern with potential role conflicts of mental health professionals — what has come to be known as the "double-agent" problem.[43] Current legal developments concerning the "right to refuse treatment" illustrate these two foci. The effort to articulate the legal and ethical limitations upon forced treatment began with suits to prevent radical procedures such as lobotomies and psychosurgery. In *Kaimowitz v. Department of Mental Health*,[44] lawyers sought to have such techniques labeled "experimental" with the object of prohibiting their use unless truly voluntary and informed consent was secured from potential subjects. Follow-up challenges on the same basis have been made to electroshock therapy, behavior modification programs employing aversive stimuli, sterilization, and, finally, to chemotherapy.

The legal theory underlying these cases is that even involuntarily committed patients have constitutional rights (e.g., the right to physical and mental privacy and autonomy or the right to protection from harm) under the First, Eighth and Fourteenth Amendments to the United States Constitution, and that these rights require limitations upon hazardous and intrusive procedures. The principle of a refusal right is perceived as all the more important when an individual's behavior has been deemed sufficiently uncontrollable or dangerous to justify involuntary civil commitment. In this latter situation, there may well be conflicts between the individual's values and behavioral goals and those of the society which has committed him. The psychiatrist or other mental health professional employed by a mental hospital or a prison may be confused as to where his primary responsibilities lie: with a particular mental patient or prisoner, with the administration of the institution which pays his salary or with the community at large.[45]

A right of mental patients to refuse treatment is difficult to articulate in theoretical terms and even more difficult to implement at the practical level. This is because informed consent, which is the traditional legal mechanism for protecting persons against unwanted intrusions into their physical or mental integrity, is often impossible for mental patients. Their illness may have rendered them incompetent to balance the risks versus benefits posed by a particular therapy and to make a treatment decision. Or a decision may not be truly voluntary, given the coercive forces inherent in institutions. As a result, many "informed consent" cases have bogged down in a conceptual morass of whether consent can ever be voluntary for a committed patient, when surrogate consent is preferable, and whether a judge or layman or even a mixed layman/professional panel's opinion on "the best interests" of the patient is superior to his doctor's.

The anticipated reaction to right-to-refuse litigation by many psychiatrists and other mental health professionals has been one of resentment against this

---

[43] See, e.g., Shestack, "Psychiatry and the Dilemmas of Dual Loyalties," *Amer. Bar Assn. Journal* 6 (1974): 1521–1524; Powledge, "The Therapist as Double Agent," *Psychology Today* (July 1977): 44–48.

[44] *Supra*, note 5.

[45] See Friedman, "Legal Regulation of Applied Behavior Analysis in Mental Institutions and Prisons," *Arizona Law Review* 17 (1975): 39, 49.

intrusion into the domain of their professional judgment. In a California case, the medical society took the position that state legislation regulating psychosurgery and electroconvulsive therapy violated a constitutionally protected private relationship between doctors and patients.[46]

To add injury to insult, two psychiatrists were recently ordered to pay personal damages to an ex-mental patient for illegally depriving him of his liberty and confining him without treatment for almost 15 years.[47] Professional indignation was forthcoming: Securing injunctive relief to improve conditions at institutions was perceived as one thing, but the American Psychiatric Association saw the move for individual civil liability as a more radical and unjustified invasion of professional discretion. The point was also made that the assessment of money damages against individual psychiatrists would drive them out of work in the public mental health system, to the great detriment of all concerned.

Contemporary professional literature is accordingly filled with hostile slogans concerning the imminent death of the mental health system from an "overdose of due process."[48] And the medical profession is beginning to mobilize to oppose both judicial reforms and legislative support for patient advocacy units.

Predictably, the efforts of legal advocates to hold psychiatrists and other mental health professionals legally accountable for their actions have been turned upon their own profession as well. Perhaps the mental health professionals who were upset by *Donaldson* have gained some measure of solace from recent legal actions seeking money damages from judges and lawyers for derelictions of their duties in mental health cases.

In 1971 an Indiana probate judge ordered the sterilization of a 15-year-old girl named Linda Sparkman, who was alleged to be mentally retarded. The petition for sterilization was presented to the defendant who appointed no guardian *ad litem* to represent Linda's interest and who issued the requested order in an *ex parte* proceeding. Years later Linda Sparkman and her husband brought an action seeking damages under the Civil Rights Act, contending that the judge's actions in ordering her sterilization violated her constitutional rights. The judge argued successfully before the United States District Court that his judicial immunity gave him absolute protection from a suit for damages. But on appeal, the Seventh Circuit reversed, finding that the purported judicial action of the defendant had no support in either state statutes or common law and that judicial immunity does not apply where a judge acts in the absence of jurisdiction.[49]

And in another case, the Wisconsin circuit court issued a scathing indictment of the shoddy legal representation given to persons who had been involuntarily

---

[46]*Doe v. Younger*, 4th Civ. No. 14407, (Cal. Ct. of Appeals, 4th Appellate District, Div. 1, April 23, 1976).

[47]The jury awarded $38,500 damages against two defendants. The Supreme Court vacated this award and remanded in *Donaldson, supra* note 8 at 577. Plaintiff eventually received a damages settlement of $20,000 in 1977.

[48]See the dissent of Judge Broderick in *Bartley v. Kremens*, 402 F. Supp. 1039, 1054 (E.D. Pa. 1975) (Three Judge Court), *vacated* and *remanded as moot*, 97 S. Ct. 1709 (1977).

[49]*Sparkman v. McFarlin*, 552 F. 2d 172 (7th Cir. 1977); As this article went to press, the Supreme Court reversed the 7th Circuit, 55 L.Ed. 2d 331, _____ U.S. _____ (1978).

committed at sham hearings.[50] In its finding, the court outlined a number of embarrassing facts; for example, only one out of nearly 1,300 cases had been tried by a jury, even though persons subject to commitment were entitled to a jury trial; the closed panel of court-appointed attorneys failed to cross-examine two out of every three witnesses against defendants and asked an average of only two questions for all witnesses; the right of persons subject to civil commitment to subpoena witnesses in their favor was waived in 99 percent of the cases; and on numerous occasions the court-appointed attorneys joined in urging commitment or detention even though their "clients" did not wish to be committed. As the circuit court wrote:

> The record presented by this case is as bleak a picture as has probably ever been presented of justice in Milwaukee County. A massive and systematic deprivation of the constitutional rights of people who are unable to voice their own protests has been accomplished by the cooperation of the bench and bar of Milwaukee County. . . . [T]he onus of the debacle lies squarely with the lawyers and judges who operated this "greased runway to the county mental health center. . . ."[51]

These cases show that with increasing litigation concerning the mental health system, at least psychiatrists, state mental health administrators, lawyers, and perhaps someday even judges, can expect to be held accountable for negligent or malicious violations of the constitutional rights of mentally handicapped persons.

In a related development, patients are asking purported advocacy groups — whether lawyers or mental health professionals or citizens — to explain why they are composed primarily of middle-class "do-gooders" but do not have in their membership a healthy proportion of actual patients or ex-patients. Again analogizing to the civil rights movement, the clients may want to take over the movement from the advocates. This move toward patient self-determination stems from several sources: a growing skepticism about the "magic" and dependability of "experts"; a disenchantment with the bureaucratization of the mental health system, which often delivers patients to impersonal civil servants working 9–5 shifts; and the politicization of civil rights movements generally, showing patients the value of lobbying, of demonstrations and of taking their cases to the legislature.

Commentary

In closing, we pause to reflect on where all this legal activity has brought us.

1. Are fewer persons being involuntarily confined who can survive on the outside without danger to others or to themselves than before this emphasis on legalism began?
2. Are more persons with identifiable mental (or socio-economic-mental) problems receiving voluntary help or treatment outside of institutions than before?

---

[50]State of Wisconsin *ex rel. David Memmel and Judith Pagels v. Mundy*, Case No. 441-417 Cir. Ct. Milwaukee County, Wisc., Aug. 18, 1976, *appeal dismissed and rights declared*, 75 Wis. 2nd 276, 249 N.W. 2d 573 (1977).

[51]*Id*. Circuit Court Sl. Op. at 15.

3. Are more people who cannot survive or who survive, but in deplorable want and mental agony, left to fend for themselves without help of any kind?
4. Are talented mental health personnel being chilled or harassed away from public service because of the legal complexities of treating anyone involuntarily or without clearly incontrovertible evidence of informed consent?
5. Are lawyer-advocates more often protecting the vulnerable from callous relatives or only isolating them from natural allies without whose kinship and kindness — no matter how ill-conceived or intermittent — they cannot survive? This is a particularly critical question with children.
6. Are stigma and discrimination against the mentally ill increasing or decreasing as a result of growing militancy?

Although we barely have a clue to the answers, the questions themselves suggest that we are confronting a conflict of values that has its roots in our United States Constitution: Which is better — liberty or the pursuit of happiness (of which mental health is an important part)?

The functions of a mental health system remain mixed in the United Sates: to treat, to protect society, to act as a last resort, to serve as a socially imposed haven for the physically and socially inept. It is unlikely these mixed goals will ever come untangled.

The tension between legal controls and mental health treatment goals will probably continue, with both sides frustrated. As long as voluntary social and mental health services continue to be inadequate in coverage and quality — as they surely will for the indefinite future; as long as mental health professionals continue not to know how to treat most patients in a way that will ensure recovery or at least improvement — as they apparently will *not* for the indefinite future; and as long as vulnerable disabled persons continue to deal inadequately with life — with their parents, their relatives, their school, work and other societal institutions — as they surely will for the indefinite future, then the mental health system has no chance of becoming pure by either the mental health or the legal standard.

The tensions among advocates — like the tensions among various branches of government or among professionals or between professionals and the consumers of mental health services — are, at least in our pluralistic system, a sign of health.

Comments on Wald and Friedman's "The Politics of Mental Health Advocacy"

Commentator: Kenneth L. Chasse*

If my comments were to have a title it would be: "The Politics of Providing Greater Access to Treatment for Those in the Criminal Justice System in Canada." We do not have in Canada, in relation to the criminal justice system and treatment of prisoners, the great disputes over policy or the great quantities of analysis necessary to resolve conflicts in principle that exist in the United States. In connection with the Mental Disorder Project of the Department of Justice, the questions that we are in the process of answering are: (a) which of these disputes and conflicts will we have? (if we recommend implementation of the recommendations of the Law Reform Commission of Canada), and (b) would we not have a healthier criminal justice system if we *did* have them? Although we do not have an extensive case law we do have a Law Reform Commission whose recommendations should be making the same issues subject to public debate. From the Canadian perspective it will be constructive to formulate comparable questions for our criminal justice system.

1. Indefinite confinement because of unfitness to stand trial – the same issue presently exists in Canada.
2. Adequate treatment is the quid pro quo for involuntary commitment – a comparable question in the criminal justice system would be, deprivation of liberty does not mean deprivation of access to treatment.
3. The "least restrictive way of treatment principle" – in the criminal justice system: a treatment principle which prevents treatment being restricted to only those who disrupt the prison system and prevents the imposition of treatment without consent if a prisoner disrupts the prison.
4. The state can create a mental health system, but if it does, that system must operate in a manner that doesn't violate rights – in the criminal justice system a comparable principle would be that if the state creates a prison system it must operate that system in a manner that doesn't violate one's access to medical treatment, including treatment for mental disability, and in a manner that provides procedural guarantees to maintain that right to access to treatment.
5. There is concern that it is the courts in the United States that are deciding how mental health resources will be allocated – in Canada this does not happen in relation to the prison system and it does not happen in the criminal justice system as a whole except for court-ordered assessments and the issue of fitness to stand trial, and indirectly through the insanity defence. We have a long way to go in Canada before we need be concerned with

---

*Special Advisor, Department of Justice, Ottawa, Canada.

over-activity in the courts' allocation of mental health facilities in regard to the criminal justice system.

6. There is concern in the United States about judicial activism from the "least powerful branch." We do not have that concern in Canada, the decision in *R. v. Boomhower* (1974) 27 C.R.N.S. 188 (O.C.A.), notwithstanding.

7. Inability to predict dangerousness justifies the civil liberties approach over the best interest of the patient, the protection of society, or the pursuit of happiness. Needless to say, the same psychiatric inability to predict dangerousness should be raising comparable issues in Canada.

8. The morale in a mental health system geared to treating the treatable will be far superior to that in one geared only to warehousing the dangerous. In relation to the Criminal Justice System one would say that morale in a prison system geared to incarcerating the hard-core professional criminal and the untreatable dangerous criminal only, will be far superior. Psychotic prisoners will be in psychiatric facilities (1 to 10% of present prison population), the first-time offenders and non-professional ineffectual offenders will be subject to non-custodial sentencing (40%), and the personality disorders will have access to treatment if both they and the psychiatric facility consent (40%). The other 10% are the hard-core professional criminals who will be left in the prisons.

9. Due process procedural protections for civil commitment: (a) prompt hearing, (b) adequate notice (c) right to retained or assigned counsel, (d) right to retained or assigned independent evaluator, (e) a transcript of the proceedings, (f) application of the principle of the least restrictive alternative, (g) a stringent standard of proof, (h) right to an expedited appeal. In Canada, it is merely argued outside the courts that there is a need for similar procedural protections to guarantee access to treatment in the criminal justice system.

10. Professional resentment of a right to refuse treatment. In Canada there is said to be professional resentment in civil psychiatric facilities of any suggestion as to treating prisoners.

11. The conflict in constitutional values between liberty and the pursuit of happiness. In Canada such issues have not yet been joined but they are coming; there is merely the behind-the-scenes conflict between the autonomy of the corrections administration in relation to treatment versus professional psychiatric independence over treatment decisions.

The Canadian Federal Department of Justice's Mental Disorder Project has been mentioned. Any project which addresses itself to these matters in relation to the criminal justice system must concern itself with three areas in relation to psychiatric services — assessment, treament, and release from treatment.

Assessment. The problems are obvious: (a) facilities, (b) professional privilege between psychiatrist and accused or inmate. There is no medical or psychiatric privilege in Canadian criminal law: there is a Federal/Provincial Task Force on Uniform Rules of Evidence looking into the problem.

Treatment. The Mental Disorder Project is evaluating the Hospital Order mechanism recommended by the Law Reform Commission, which gives the trial judge power to consider ordering treatment for a person sentenced to imprisonment — but only after sentence is imposed *and* only if the accused *and* the psychiatric facility consent.

Release from Treatment. We are (a) re-evaluating the Lieutenant Governor's Warrant which allows for confinement of mentally ill prisoners, those found unfit to stand trial, and those found not guilty by reason of insanity; (b) re-evaluating the Cabinet's power over release from the Lieutenant Governor's Warrant, (c) re-evaluating the procedures of our Review Boards which supervise those Lieutenant Governor's Warrants and make recommendations to the Cabinet.

Should release of mentally ill prisoners be by (a) Cabinet decision, or (b) commitment under Civil Mental Health legislation, or (c) by an expert board which is subject to judicial review and required to give reasons and provide other procedural guarantees to decision making? In the event that we legislate any of these alternatives, we may expect to produce the type of case law that Patricia Wald and Paul Friedman have reviewed.

In dealing with problems in relation to guaranteeing adequate access to treatment for prisoners, the main issues that the Mental Disorder Project has isolated in consultations with psychiatric colleagues in the western provinces have included:

1. *The Hospital order and the right to treatment:* the hospital order mechanism would require the recognition *in effect* of a right which does not presently exist — the right of the prisoner to access to treatment (regulations 2.06 and 3.05 under the Penitentiaries Act notwithstanding).
2. *Treatment of personality disorders:* such right will allow prisoners to call for treatment of not only psychoses but personality disorders as well.
3. *Parity of treatment:* such right must not give greater access to treatment than that enjoyed by the general population, i.e., it must provide for regional disparity.
4. *Impact on psychiatric facilities:* ascertaining the percentage of prison populations suffering personality disorders — we have received estimates from 20 to 80%; those suffering psychoses from 1 to 10%.
5. *Adequacy of existing facilities:* no jurisdiction has psychiatric facilities sufficient to treat even a substantial fraction of prisoner personality disorders.
6. *Administrative vs. judicial mechanisms:* the question as to whether personality disorders can be treated through administrative mechanisms rather than creating a judicial mechanism called a "hospital order" must be answered; in theory it can be, but numerous commission and government reports have shown that it just doesn't happen (see the *1913 Royal Commission Investigation into the Insane Ward at Kingston Penitentiary,* the *Archambault Report* of 1938, the *Fauteux Report* of 1958, the *Commissioner of Penitentiaries Report* of 1969, and the *Report to Parliament by the Sub-*

Committee on the Penitentiary System in Canada, 1977).

7. *Present plan for building forensic psychiatric facilities:* generally, present building plans look to treating the psychotic, but only experimenting with treatment of the personality disorder.

8. *The variety in Canadian mental health systems:* federal proposals for treating prisoners will have to be tailored to fit each province, and in some cases different parts of the same province.

9. *Professional staffing of psychiatric facilities:* psychiatrists are generally in short supply; those interested in forensic psychiatry are a small minority; of them an even smaller minority believes there is reason to hope for success in treating personality disorders.

10. *Incompatibility between the approach taken by civil psychiatric facilities and the treatment of personality disorders:* the treatment of psychoses is well-defined, amenable to drug therapy, short, and therefore compatible with treatment in civil psychiatric facilities or possibly right in the prison; the treatment of personality disorders is not well-defined, it is measured in years, it must look to behavioral modification rather than chemical therapy and it is said to be completely incompatible with the practices of civil psychiatric units or prisons.

11. *Resistance by civil facilities to taking in the prisoner personality disorder:* we are told by forensic psychiatrists that civil psychiatric facilities resist treating the personality disorder; they lack experience with prisoners' particular psychiatric problems; they find them disruptive; prisoner personality disorders are incompatible with the present strong commitment to short-term hospitalization and "community psychiatry"; civil psychiatric units fear the repercussions from mixing civil patients with prisoners. The opinion we have received from psychiatrists is that one cannot hope to use civil psychiatric facilities despite the fact that dwindling mental populations represent unused capacity and lay-offs. One needs psychiatrists trained in the particular problems of criminals and prisoners. Regardless of how much the resistance of civil psychiatric facilities may be an attitudinal incompatibility rather than an actual or real incompatibility there is nonetheless a formidable body of resistance.

12. *Facilities that have to be built:* if existing civil facilities cannot be used we must ascertain what additional forensic psychiatric facilities will have to be built.

13. *The conflict between the psychiatrist and the prison administration:* treatment of personality disorders requires a "therapeutic community"; such may be incompatible with a corrections or prison atmosphere and administrative approach. There may be a way of having the advantages of both models by providing sufficient guarantees of effective input by psychiatrists into administrative decision-making in regard to admittance, treatment, discharge and the handling of prisoners while undergoing treatment — perhaps administrative rules or contract provisions backed-up with effective enforcement.

14. *Return to prison after treatment:* psychiatrists are very reluctant to accept long-term prisoners for treatment if the completion of treatment means a return to prison which will undo the treatment; yet it is the long-term pris-

oner who is most likely to have the severest psychiatric disorder and the longest record. Therefore, mechanisms guaranteeing input by psychiatrists into the decision-making process in regard to how the remainder of a sentence is to be served after treatment must be developed or sentence-shortening considered.

15. *Sentence-shortening:* the sensitive issue of sentence-shortening on successful completion of treatment must be answered. If the psychiatric cause of the crime is removed, should not the sentence be shortened once treatment is successfully completed? Will a parole board, a board of psychiatrists, a review board, or the judge shorten the sentence? Preliminary indications are that the majority of judges do not want to get into sentence supervision, but is the issue not too important to be left entirely to the opinion of the judiciary?

16. *Hospital orders while sentence is being served, after the imposition of sentence:* if the convicted are to be guaranteed access to treatment by being able to apply for a hospital order at the time of imposing sentence, should there not be a similar guarantee while sentence is being served? What type of body must be put in place to guarantee proper consideration of a prisoner's application for transfer to a psychiatric facility, and later, for transfer back to the prison?

17. *Estimating the impact of treatment upon psychiatric facilities:* estimating what impact the making of treatment available for personality disorders will have upon psychiatric facilities can be done in only general terms. Precision forecasting is not possible since, for example, psychiatrists themselves do not agree upon what personality disorders are in need of treatment.

18. *The limited hospital order:* if initially, a hospital order mechanism is enacted which limits the types of disorder open to treatment because of the uncertainty of the impact (upon existing facilities and the quantity of new facilities needed), can a dividing line be drawn which will not be seen to be arbitrary and unjust and which will not aggravate the present disparity in sentencing and in the handling of prisoners?

19. *Support programs to reduce the impact on hospital orders:* diversion programs and alternatives-to-sentencing programs for those in the criminal justice system suffering psychiatric disorders must be developed in conjunction with the hospital order so as to minimize the impact that the hospital order will have upon psychiatric facilities. The hospital order is available only on imposing a sentence of imprisonment; if there is no other way of securing treatment, judges may sentence to imprisonment in order to get access to the hospital order and the length of sentence may be made to fit the anticipated needs of treatment.

20. *Consent to treatment:* if consent to treatment by convicted persons before the court on sentencing or by inmates is to be a key feature of any treatment program or statutory mechanism, who will determine if they have the capacity to give an informed and voluntary consent? Is this a new function that can be given to existing review boards?

21. *Using unused capacity in psychiatric facilities:* can unused psychiatric facilities be taken over for the treatment of prisoners? Populations of mental institutions are dwindling; an inventory of all psychiatric facilities is neces-

sary; can we expect the taxpayer to support the building of new facilities when hospitals are being closed and psychiatric workers are suffering lay offs?

22. *An honest foundation in principle for justifying increased access to treatment:* what is the correct principle upon which to put forward to the public the idea of increased access to treatment for prisoners? It is not intellectually honest to say at this time that psychiatric treatment will reduce crime, although common sense may suggest that it must; studies have not been done in Canada comparing treated and non-treated groups of released prisoners as to recidivism. Also, to argue that by treatment one can reduce crime requires that one give assurances as to being able to predict future dangerousness of treated inmates, and psychiatrists acknowledge that their art has not developed that ability sufficiently in order to give such assurances. The idea of increased treatment may have to be presented as simply being the right thing to do; if we deprive a man of his freedom we should not deprive him of his access to psychiatric treatment, just as we would not think of depriving him of treatment for physical ailments by means of imprisonment. This is compatible with a presently popular view that prison without treatment does not rehabilitate, that it does not make one a penitent in a penitentiary, and that it is destructive and criminogenic.

23. *Foreign experience to be evaluated:* the experience of other countries in treating prisoners and personality disorders must be examined to avoid making the mistakes they have learned to remedy.

24. *The procedures used by Canadian Review Boards:* the present practices of review boards must be examined; what are their procedures? Should they have the final decision on release rather than the Cabinet? Should "due process" models bringing courtroom rules of procedure be imposed upon them? Can they provide guarantees reflective of the increased interest in prisoners' rights? Do their decisions mean Lieutenant-Governor's Warrants result in unjust indeterminate sentences?

25. *Confinement under Lieutenant-Governor's Warrants:* is the Lieutenant-Governor's Warrant still necessary for the successful plea of insanity? What impact would a hospital order mechanism have upon the frequency of pleas of insanity? Or upon the claims of unfitness to stand trial due to insanity or other mental illness? Is it too early to advocate that success on a plea of insanity should mean complete release from the criminal justice sytem without control unless the controls of the mental health system apply?

26. *The danger of raising expectations:* we have been warned that new programs for the treatment of prisoners can create unfulfilled expectations which lead to suicides in prisons and the sudden appearance of more mental disorder than was previously thought to exist; and also to an expectation of perfect cures and solutions for crime amongst the public.

Only when we begin improving access to treatment for prisoners and recognizing what, in effect, will be a right of access to treatment and the comparable procedural safeguards to decision-making, will we see problems reflected in our case law that are comparable to those presented in the Wald and Friedman's paper.

Comments on Wald and Friedman's "The Politics of Mental Health Advocacy"

Commentator: Mr. Justice Horace Krever*

Frankly, I approached this paper looking for a basis for challenging the writers. I was disappointed that I found none. More particularly, the conflicting positions were so fairly stated that I was unable to discern the authors' bias. It may be, I thought, that the explanation was that each author had a conflicting bias. The point I am trying to make is that the subject being discussed, the politics (with a small "p" and in the respectable sense of the word) of mental health advocacy, is a subject upon which every person has a bias of one kind or another. I certainly had one and I would be intellectually dishonest if I suggested that the bias was erased by judicial appointment. My bias, I candidly admit, was toward civil-liberties. I believe strongly in the importance of freedom and in the deplorability of the deprivation of liberty. That is not to say that I do not agree that, in some circumstances, the deprivation of liberty, however generally deplorable, may be unavoidable. The dilemma, for me, is the difficulty of articulating with certainty what those circumstances are in a way which circumscribes as much as possible the power of others to deprive me of my liberty.

Before I comment on some of the problems canvassed in Wald and Friedman's paper, as they arise in a Canadian setting, I want to digress briefly to point out a few differences between the context of the issues in the United States and Canada. Perhaps the most fundamental difference is the overwhelming and pervasive part played in any examination of these difficult questions by constitutional considerations in the United States. An almost equally patent difference is the extent to which the fight has been fought in the United States in the courts of the land. The forum here has been not judicial but legislative. Whether this will always be the case is not easy to say but I believe it can be safely predicted that the competition of ideas will not take the form of constitutional arguments in the American sense, that is to say arguments based on the written constitution of the nation. It is not as easy to predict that some of the issues will not be brought before our courts, however.

Whatever the differences in forum, the issues are common to both countries. In what I am about to say about civil commitment I shall use Ontario as my model, because I am naturally more familiar with my own province. In Canada, of course, civil commitment, unlike the criminal process about which Mr. Chasse will speak and which is a federal matter, is within the exclusive legislative jurisdiction of the provincial legislatures, as being part of property and civil rights in the province. There is a current controversy about this very subject, a controversy having its origin in proposals to amend *The Mental Health Act,* now

*Supreme Court of Ontario, Canada. Justice Krever is Commissioner of the Royal Commission of Enquiry into the Confidentiality of Health Records in Ontario.

Chapter 269 of the Revised Statutes of Ontario 1970, but enacted only some 10 years ago, in 1967, as chapter 51. Time will not permit an exhaustive description of the provisions of the statute as it reads today but I think it important that I refer to the current legislative criteria for involuntary admission to a psychiatric facility:

> 7. Any person who is believed to be in need of the observation, care and treatment provided in a psychiatric facility may be admitted thereto as an informal patient upon the recommendation of a physician.

> 8. (1) Any person who,
>> (a) suffers from mental disorder of a nature or degree so as to require hospitalization in the interests of his own safety or the safety of others; and
>> (b) is not suitable for admission as an informal patient,
> may be admitted as an involuntary patient to a psychiatric facility upon application therefor in the prescribed form signed by a physician.

> (2) It shall be stated and shown clearly that the physician signing the application personally examined the person who is the subject of the application and made due inquiry into all of the facts necessary for him to form a satisfactory opinion.

> (3) The physician signing the application shall also in the application state the facts upon which he has formed his opinion of the mental disorder, distinguishing the facts observed by him from the facts communicated to him by others, and shall note the date upon which the examination was made.

> (4) Every such application shall be completed no later than seven days after the examination referred to therein, and no person shall be admitted to a psychiatric facility upon an application except within fourteen days of the date on which the application was completed.

> (5) Such an application is sufficient authority,
>> (a) to any person to convey the person who is the subject of the application to a psychiatric facility; and
>> (b) to the authorities thereof to admit and detain him therein for a period of not more than one month.

Note that the application is authority for detaining the patient for not more than one month. By section 13, that detention may be extended by a certificate of renewal by the attending physician using the same criteria as for the initial commitment. The certificate of renewal operates as authority to detain the patient for not more than two additional months, in the case of a first certificate, not more than three additional months in the case of a second certificate, not more than six additional months in the case of a third certificate and for each subsequent certificate for not more than twelve additional months each. An involuntary patient may, under section 28 of the Act, appeal to a review board against his or her detention when any certificate of renewal comes into force.

In recent months *The Mental Health Act* has come under considerable criticism from public interest groups and particularly from the Canadian Civil Liberties Association. In March 1977 that association presented a brief to the Minister of Health in which it referred to some empirical evidence, and legal opinions relating to that evidence, of a large number of certificates committing patients to psychiatric facilities that were not properly completed and that failed to satisfy the requirements of the Act. It was said that 70% of the 200 certificates studied "violated the minimum safeguards" of the Act. Now, it must be pointed out that the point that was made was not that the 140 persons who were committed, or whose commitment was renewed, ought not to have been committed or ought not to have had their commitment renewed or were not, in fact, certifiable, but only that they ought not to have been committed or to have had their commitment renewed on the strength of the certificates that were completed. Among the five recommendations made by the Association were the following three.

1. Such commitments shall require that the person involved suffer from a mental disorder of such a nature that there is a high probability he will imminently cause, himself or someone else, serious physical injury.
2. Physicians' certificates authorizing involuntary commitment shall be limited to emergency periods of no more than 72 hours.
3. Involuntary commitments beyond such 72 hour periods shall require review by an independent official or tribunal.

Following the submission of that brief there was introduced in the Legislature (which prorogued before the bill was passed so that the bill will have to be dealt with at the next session) a bill amending *The Mental Health Act.* If enacted, section 8 will be repealed and the following language will be substituted for it. I will not reproduce all of it.

8. (1) Where a physician examines a person and has reason to believe that the person,
    (a) has threatened or attempted or is threatening or attempting to cause bodily harm to himself;
    (b) has behaved or is behaving violently towards another person or has caused or is causing another person to fear bodily harm from him; or
    (c) has shown or is showing a lack of competence to care for himself,
    and the physician is of the opinion that the person is apparently suffering from mental disorder of a nature or quality that likely will result in,
    (d) serious bodily harm to the person;
    (e) serious bodily harm to another person; or,
    (f) imminent and serious physical impairment of the person,

the physician may make application in the prescribed form for a psychiatric assessment of the person

*   *   *

(5) An application under subsection 1 is sufficient authority for seven days from and including the day on which it is signed by the physician,

    (a) to a person to take the person who is the subject of the application in custody to a psychiatric facility; and

    (b) to detain the person who is the subject of the application in a psychiatric facility and to restrain, observe, examine and care for him in the facility for not more than 72 hours.

Furthermore, section 13 will be repealed in part. Under the new scheme, where a person is detained under section 8 the attending physician, after observing and examining the patient, must discharge him from the psychiatric facility if he is of the opinion that he is not in need of treatment or,

    13. (1) Where a person is detained under section 8 or 25, the attending physician, after observing and examining the person,

*   *   *

    (c) shall admit the person as an involuntary patient by completing and filing with the officer in charge a certificate of involuntary admission if the attending physician is of the opinion both that the person is suffering from mental disorder of a nature or quality that likely will result in,

        (i) serious bodily harm to the person,

        (ii) serious bodily harm to another person, or

        (iii) imminent and serious physical impairment of the person,

unless the person remains in the custody of a psychiatric facility and that the person is not suitable for admission as an informal patient.

A further provision of interest is the following:

    13. (3) The officer in charge shall release a person who is detained under section 8 or 25 upon the completion of 72 hours of such detention unless the attending physician has released the person, has admitted the person as an informal patient or has admitted the person as an involuntary patient by completing and filing with the officer in charge a certificate of involuntary admission.

Finally for present purposes, the periods of detention under the various certificates have been drastically curtailed. They are two weeks for the first, one additional month under a first certificate of renewal, 2 under a second, and 3 under all subsequent certificates of renewal.

No comment is necessary on the relationship between public interest lobbying (again in the best sense of the word) and legislative change. The reaction to the proposed change was predictable. The very arguments reflected in Wald and Friedman's paper are raging on all sides at this very moment. My impression is that editorial comment in the popular press is favorable. According to the press, the reaction of the Ontario Psychiatric Association, or a spokesman for it, is hostile and suggestive of a developing reluctance, if not refusal, by psychiatrists to certify persons who should be certified out of a fear of legal liability. In turn, that reaction has spawned criticism of the "psychiatric profession" at large by Mental Health/Ontario, a division of the Canadian Mental Health Association or a spokesman for it. Nevertheless, it is not unlikely that these changes will be enacted.

Behind the legislation, however, lies the really difficult problem, Civil commitment involves or presupposes the ability to predict future behavior and it is this aspect of the matter, as Wald and Friedman bring out well, that is, and I think should be, the cause of concern. Psychiatric literature does not provide the basis for overconfidence in the state of the art of psychiatric diagnosis or of competence to predict dangerous or violent behavior. It seems to me that a stronger case can be made for confining a member of society in a place of safety by reason of the commission of a past harmful act than for a predicted act which, in truth, may never occur. In any event, however strong the case for committing one who is a threat to the safety of others, from the point of view of political or social philosophy, is the case as strong for doing so in the case of a threat to one's self? It may not be entirely out of place to recall that it was not that many years ago that the offence of attempted suicide was removed from the Canadian Criminal Code, or in modern jargon, was "decriminalized." In other areas of health policy, after all, society does not act so paternalistically — for example, in the use of tobacco and alcohol which, in both cases, is demonstrably inimical to health.

Two other points deserve brief mention. The first is the problem of compulsory treatment in the context of the usual requirement of informed consent of the patient. The debate on this subject may soon become as heated here as it has in the United States. It will be recalled that the proposed new legislation provides that the application is "sufficient authority . . . to detain the person who is the subject of the application in a psychiatric facility and to *restrain, observe, examine and care for him* in the facility for not more than 72 hours." Similar authority is conferred by a certificate of involuntary admission under the proposed new section 13 as well as by certificates of renewal. Whether that statutory language will be interpreted as abolishing the need for the patient's consent is, I suppose, a potential problem, but inherent in the whole question of mental illness is the eternal dilemma of the importance of the absence of consent where the need for treatment is present and the patient, if competent, refuses to consent, or, if incompetent, cannot consent. The validity of surrogate consent by a committee or other person has never been satisfactorily determined. Finally, I mention, but only mention (because of my current preoccupation with the problem in more than a philosophical way on a royal commission of enquiry) the difficult issue of the confidentiality of psychiatric histories and records and access by patients to their own records.

The Mask of Psychopathy

Ole Nygaard Jensen*

During its almost 200 year history, psychopathy has been of much concern to the public. The concept of psychopathy has caused much trouble and frustration to scientists, and the so-called psychopath has given an exhausting amount of work to those dealing with the treatment of psychopathy. Psychiatrists seemingly have not been able to convey their conception of psychopathy to the public. We are all familiar with the misuse of the word psychopath for a dislikable person. Furthermore, in recent years we have experienced a strong interest in the so-called political dissidents and their relation to psychiatry. From a platform of practical experience, being responsible for the institutional treatment and correction of persons suffering from psychopathy, it is my firm opinion that the ghost of psychopathy is to be found in the midst of the problem of the so-called political misuse of psychiatry. However, it seems to me that it is public opinion and its spokesmen, the politicians, that are misusing psychiatry. We are witnessing a curiously political and unholy alliance between the reactionary right wing and the bewildered part of the left wing uniting in their furious attack on psychiatry.

To psychiatrists it is well known that a form of psychopathy may be expressed in a rigid, all-absorbing criticism of systems. It is not the criticism of the system that is in itself wrong. The way in which you criticize decides whether you are normal, psychopathic or psychotic. It is the responsibility of the psychiatrist, sometimes in collaboration with the judge, to make this decision with due respect to the specific culture, the law and the individual life story. It is not the membership in a subculture nor the violation of the law, nor the fact that one is a peculiar personality, that creates the impression of psychopathy. The concept of psychopathy deals in its core with morality, guilt and love. However, it is not the specific morals of the psychiatrist or the judge that are decisive; neither is it the specific morals of the society, all of which are contaminants that must be removed before you can see the lack of morality in psychopathy. Every once in a while the psychiatrists themselves contribute to the confusion around the concept of psychopathy, as for example when McCord and McCord claimed that psychopathy constituted a threat to the American way of life.[1] But to be fair, they also said that any adequate study of psychopathy must look beyond asociality.

Since psychiatry, as well as being a control system of social deviancy also pretends to be a science, I am compelled as a psychiatrist to clarify some impor-

---

*Senior Psychiatrist, Herstedvester Treatment Center, Copenhagen, Denmark.
[1]McCord and McCord, *The Psychopath, An Essay on the Criminal Mind* (New York: Van Nostrand Reinhold, 1964).

tant points about the concept of psychopathy. I do not want to give a definition of psychopathy, but rather wish to discuss morality and immorality. I will
describe the psychopath as a public mythological figure viewed in his brotherhood with "the regular guy," and then explore the problem of a psychological
theory of psychopathy.

On Morality

Morality treats the relations between people in a society. It deals with the
engagements and the responsibility that we feel to the social contracts that we
enter into with other people. The solidarity that we confirm in being confronted with another person — beyond the singular moment and the singular situation, confirms us mutually in our identity as human beings and individualities
in a concrete historical society. This is the definition of social contracts which
are displayed in small and large relations every day. Morality is something we
learn through social contracts as soon as we have a language to learn with. We
learn morality by means of our acts, which are behaviors seen in the context of
their objective social results. Of course the little baby has not yet entered as a
human being this world of morality and guilt.

Breach of contract, breach of confidence does move us deeply. We become
distressed and angry. When we disregard a social contract, we feel guilty. We
have acted immorally. Whenever we meet an individual who disregards a confidence, an agreement or a social contract, we expect to find stamps of guilt on
this person. If we do find the marks of guilt, we can forgive, because we are
then confirmed in our identity, in our belief in the validity of the social contract. The other person is guilty and immoral, but after all human.

It is essential in our concept of psychopathy and the psychopathic person
that he significantly fails in an I-thou relationship in the way that he behaves
immorally and without feelings of guilt. If it was only about a deviance from
the morals, the norms and standards of the given society, quite a number of
people with high morality and outstanding capacity for solidarity would be
numbered as being psychopaths — for instance people who oppose strongly the
politically established system of society.

The concept of psychopathy deals primarily with a missing morality and guilt,
with a lacking capacity for solidarity in I-thou relationships, with being "non-
human," which is to deny the other person the confirmation of his identity as a
human being. Secondarily this deficit, which we characterize as an insufficiency
or defect of the personality, often will lead to antisocial behavior.

These words about morality and immorality in fact reflect the whole psychopathology of psychopathy. It would be more precise to speak of amorality
rather than immorality when defining psychopathy, since the immorality implies a knowledge and an acceptance of morality, which is outside the range
and understanding of the person exhibiting psychopathy. As Hobbes put it:
"The wicked man is but the child grown strong." We do face a man called the
psychopath, who is a lonely wolf, highly impulsive, a victim of his own immediate desires, unable to form lasting bonds of affection with other human beings. Although this psychopath seemingly speaks the language, he is suffering

from what Cleckley calls "semantic dementia" and may be viewed as a reflex machine, imitating a normal human being.

What is important to notice when we talk about morality is the central position of the language in the division between what is moral and human and what is amoral and thereby "non-human." But when we switch to the language of psychopathology something happens: the language turns from being dynamic and concerned about interhuman relations into a static, individual-centered language, and we have created the psychopath. The psychopath is popularly viewed as a monster in line with the Frankenstein monster. In my practice I have never met a concrete person that could be described as such a "psychopath monster." On the other hand it is my daily work to deal with psychopathy displayed by real persons. The problem is that while criminologists and behavioral scientists are counting psychopathy in numbers of psychopaths, the psychiatrists are dealing with real "here and now" persons that frequently are captured in a peculiar form of communication that may be described as psychopathy. But the psychiatrists are also prisoners of the individual-centered language and its linkage to the world of public mythology, which I can best illustrate with the language of a case story.

Case History: Kaj

Kaj is 45 years old and has been, since early youth, under institutional care, later having been both in reformatories and prisons, owing to an increasing number of offences, mainly check forgeries. He grew up in economically stable circumstances, but was very split, especially by his father, who weakened to many of Kaj's demands, although his mother attempted to be resolute and consistent in his upbringing. Kaj's own thoughts were that his mother was quite steadfast and somewhat strict. As he was the only son he was favored at the expense of his sisters, with the result that he had no duties in the home. In adult life he married, but this only lasted for a short time and since then he has never been involved in a long-standing relationship. Kaj never succeeded in getting any education as such and was always very restless and unstable in any work situation. Restlessness and excitement are actually what make him tick, although from time to time he finds it an exhausting way to live.

During his numerous incarcerations, those who have been in contact with him have described him as extremely moody and unpredictable. He can be very friendly and good-natured, but is unable to cope with adverse circumstances and cannot bear the rejection of any request. He is very self-centered and is referred to as being thoroughly unreliable in all respects: even his fellow prisoners have a hard time dealing with him. His behavior toward his superiors, at work and in prison, can change from that of crying, whimpering, despairing, full of self-pity, to condescending arrogance and self-confidence ending in primitive and rude behavior. He has no insight or self-criticism, although he at times may give as the explanation of his

restless way of living and his criminality, that he is too gifted and in-
telligent and that his brain is functioning too fast. It is evident that
in such situations he firmly believes his own statements.

Kaj may be happy and excited like a child, when he is out shopping and is getting help of various kinds to obtain social goods. But,
in spite of his seemingly wholehearted participation in rehabilitation,
everything goes to pieces in a short time, the process starting almost
immediately after his release. It is a characteristic trait, that when
Kaj wants something (which he does quite often and without propor-
tionality), he is not able to listen to arguments or realistic application
of the brakes. He seems to be in an eternal quest for affirmative answers. At times he may be worried and anxious about himself and his
future. He may then be somewhat confused and bewildered and feels
like a man from Mars in his relations with other people.

During a serious illness he refused to accept the indispensable treatment. He wanted to take the chance of dying in a normal way from a
disease, and he found this to be an exciting game and remained unaf-
fected by the fact that he was playing with his own life. Frequently
he would seize the slightest occasion to quarrel about trivialities in
the medical treatment.

He sets forth assertions and plans that are utterly unfounded. For
example he once worked hard to get a typewriter and writing paper
with his own name printed on it, because, as he explained, he had received an order for a theatrical play for television. He insisted on this
and referred to his connections at the national TV center. At last we
came to the core of the matter, which was a friendly talk he had had
with an engineer from the TV center. During their conversation Kaj
out of a sudden impulse told the engineer about a plan for a theatrical play, – and while Kaj was talking and explaining the engineer several times murmured: "yes, yes."

Comments: This story sounds like the story of a psychopath, but it should
be read as a description of psychopathy. Living together with Kaj has taught
me about moments of despair, hope and fear for the future, that openly express
a knowledge of the language of the others, the language of responsible meaning.
Psychopathy is not a static quality of a person, but a dynamic form of communication, which implies that treatment (i.e., change) is possible.

The Psychopath: a Public Myth

While I have to respect the reality of psychopathy I cannot accept the notion of the psychopath except as being a mythological figure. You may accuse
me of quibbling, but the hair-splitting is as important to me as the difference
between a mediate scientific language and an immediate language unconsciously contaminated with ideologies and myths, that present themselves as if they
represented reality. The immediate language of public opinion is populated by
fetish-figures that all have their specific function within our culture bound universe.

When you force the experience of psychopathy into the body of a real person you have created a self-fulfilling prophecy, the psychopath, who is in the negative mirroring the "regular guy," the normal well-behaving bourgeois. The psychopath is the evil, the cruel one, the freebooter, who is not bound by the standing rules of society or by interhuman engagements. The attitude of the bourgeois public toward this figure is highly ambivalent. He is glorified as the lonely hero, who disengages our dreams about a limitless freedom, and then dreaded (and rejoiced in) because of his cruel (often sexual) actions.

The psychopath is intimately related in a brotherhood with the bourgeois myth about the normal citizen as the wicked and the good son. The figure supplements an important scapegoat function of public utility, which, however, at the same time fills up the position of the real person. As the idea of the mythological figure, the psychopath also embodies the normal, good citizen, an ideological myth. They are both a product of history. The normal, good citizen is a child of the bourgeois revolution, that raised the idea of man as an autonomous individual born with an innate free will. In this way the psychopath figure became the reflected, negative image of the bourgeois, who under inward struggle and deprivation has had to renounce his natural free will and autonomous freedom in the interests of the society in opposition to the psychopath, who takes unlawful liberties and freedom. The psychopath becomes the caricature of the bourgeois saying: everyone is the maker of his own fate. But for both of them it is a game of illusion around the conception of freedom and liberty. First, when you realize that the essence of man is to be found in the total context of social relations, it is possible to perceive that freedom is not a natural quality or an individual property. Social relations are at root nothing other than relations between people. Freedom refers to the mutual connections and solidarity among people. In fact, freedom is the acknowledged necessity.

In a cruel logical way the psychopath being himself a myth reflects the bourgeois universe of mythology. In describing his eventual longings for the future he pictures a family, in itself an ideal autonomous unit, with himself as an independent property owner or an independent skilled worker (driver of a motorvan is a preferred job), a couple of polite children and a neat home-working housewife. If you dig into his idea of the woman, you will find the common two-faced figure of the madonna and the whore with no mark of a real woman. He himself being a man depicts his father figure either as a vague trace, a cipher or as a stern, strict, but just man.

This reminds us of the phenomenon of the "double expectations" described by Stürup.[2] The influence of the "double expectations" makes the psychopath perceive any type of attitude toward him by other persons as based on their supposed constant awareness of him as a psychopath, and as such likely to react differently from "normal" fellow-citizens. In other words, if you are viewing and describing psychopathy from the position of the "regular guy," you have then created the psychopath," who is willing to fulfill all your wishes.

This intimate brotherhood may display itself within a family and even within the life story of a single individual as illustrated in the following case story:

---

[2]Georg K. Stürup, *Treating the "Untreatable"* (Baltimore: Johns Hopkins Press, 1968).

Erik is a 39 year-old man, who was raised in an ordinary petit-bourgeois home. He has not much to tell about his parents, whom he describes as being nice and normal people. He vaguely suggests that the father was a very strict, but also a rather absent person, whereas the mother was a mild and good natured woman. In the same way the parents on their side have had nothing peculiar or characteristic to tell about Erik, whom they describe as a quiet, honest, truthful and trustworthy boy, who never created any problems during his up-bringing. During his childhood and youth he never was in bad company and drank and smoked modestly. He was always very tidy, meticulous and careful about himself as well as about his things and his work. During long periods he preferred to stay by himself with absolutely no interest in company. At his working place he was reserved and had no special contact with his fellow workers. Because of his special job as an engineer it was possible for him only to have minimal contact with others. He had an excellent career within his field, with steady and prolonged employment.

Erik's wife describes him as being moody and insecure, but ambitious — a climber holding his own. He is very vulnerable and sensitive to what other people think about him. He is also said to be considerate and a willing helper. In the area of sex he admits to being immature and inexperienced. He clearly looks upon sex as being something bad and disgusting. He feels physical dislike when women flirt. He may feel the same strong distaste in other situations of a "non-sexual" character when he experiences people forcing themselves emotionally upon him, or even if they just use a more direct form of contact than the one he is able to use. He holds in considerable contempt most of his fellow-beings and seeks to avoid their company.

A sudden change in behavior occured in connection with his divorce of 10 years ago. The divorce was a quiet affair, which was initiated by his wife. She felt they had grown apart. At the same time he was involved in a minor inaccuracy in his accounts, which led to a lawsuit. To his uttermost bewilderment he lost the case. He was not able to understand it. He felt as if all the justice and values of the society had been suddenly drawn away from him. As in a revelation it was disclosed to him that in the eyes of the other beings he might be the fool, a role which he had reserved exclusively for others.

Erik then started his criminal career "for the sake of gain," armed robbery and violent acts. He has been imprisoned several times. He explains that his crimes give him at the moment of action a certain stimulating feeling of excitement and a feeling of relief and triumph. It is interesting to note that during an armed robbery Erik wounded an innocent person, just because this person was drunk and did not behave well. He had no remorse for this unnecessary act of violence, which he justified on the basis of the inappropriate behavior and disgusting drunkenness of the unlucky person. Except for the above mentioned moments of excitement, relief and triumph he is constantly depressed and often thinks of committing suicide. He holds himself and his criminal acts in much contempt.

Comment: This story, which is not an outstanding example, may illustrate how the "normality" and seemingly social sanity in the name of the "regular guy" is masking psychopathy.

On Theory

It is well known that to date we have no consistent psychological theory of psychopathy. We have several common sense hypotheses, but there is no consensus about them and they are not part of a consistent theory. It is amazing to face the fact that psychoanalysis does not mention psychopathy. Alexander's theory about the neurotic character is the closest we come to a scientific approach to our problem.[3] Alexander advises us to read the acts of the psychopath in the same way as we read the symptoms of the neurotic. The difference between the two is then to be found in a sort of "geographical" difference, namely that the symptoms of the psychopath take place in the "environment" while the symptoms of the neurotic take place in the "inner psychic life" and in somatic symptoms of the singular body. But this tells us nothing new and leads us nowhere in our dilemma. Again we are caught in the web of the individual-centered language that hides the ideology of human relations as being something that exists prior to social relations.

We clearly recognize that the psychology of the animal is different from that of man. The psychology of the animal is essentially predetermined by a biologically inherited patrimony, which is not the case with the psychology of man. When we speak about morality we are saying that psychopathy in a way is to be nonhuman. Does this then mean that the psychopath is an animal? No, it does not. But we may come dangerously close to saying so, if we deal with a concept of man and human relations as a given object that can be read and understood outside the context of social relations.

But this was exactly what happened to our most prominent theory of human personality, psychoanalysis, when it was exported to North America and re-exported to Western Europe. Psychoanalysis in practice turned out to be an ego-psychology and thereby strengthened and preserved the bourgeois idea of man. Our psychology seems to have given a "role" to history, society or "environment." But on the contrary, we may state through analysis that history has produced our psychology and has given it a role in preserving the given power structures in our culture.

However, if we read the Freudian psychoanalysis carefully we may find that the theory first of all is a frontal attack on the idea of man being an autonomous individual equipped with independent character traits, free will and freedom. Through the description of the unconscious, psychoanalysis has contributed to the understanding of man and human relations. But the unconscious itself should be analyzed and understood in the context of social relations. One

---

[3] Frantz Alexander, "The Neurotic Character" (1930): *Int. Journal Psycho-Anal.* 292–311.

cannot explain history from the unconscious. My personality is part of history. The unconscious itself is part of history.

We have to realize that the reason we do not have a psychological theory of psychopathy is because we do not have a theory of human personality. And this is true both for bourgeois and socialist cultures, since Marxism does not deal with the theory of human personality in the sense of a study of concrete individuals, and social psychology has not dealt with the problem of the unconscious. On the other hand, a science of psychology that is not based on historical materialism is damned to remain in the haze of idealism, in its futile attempt to create a given object that has something to do with reality. When founding the science of history, Marx totally rejected the project of constructing a given object, e.g., a general abstract model of all society viewing each specific society as a variant of the model. Instead he approached society as the processes of production and reproduction of social life.

Marx taught us that the individual is a product of history, not of nature. This means that human beings, viewed as developed personalities, are produced by social relations and that a natural general form of human individuality has never existed anywhere. Every social formation has at once its characteristic social relations and its specific forms of human individuality. Thus the specific forms of human individuality in the feudal society are different from the forms of human individuality which we find in the capitalistic, bourgeois society. This important point has been documented in a beautiful way in the works of Michel Foucault. But this also means that psychopathy, as it is personified and acted out by the person we call the psychopath, is to be viewed as a specific form of human individuality intimately related to the specific social relations that characterize the capitalistic, bourgeois society. Furthermore, this also implies that psychopathy has a different meaning in a capitalistic than a socialist society. In a socialist society psychopathy is bound to take the major form of a "system criticism," because it is a reactionary "system criticism" closely related to the bourgeois figure and his system. Having liberated the concrete person from living under the yoke of being a mythological figure, the psychopath, we must state that psychopathy is not a blue fog disconnected from reality. Psychopathy refers to acts performed by concrete persons and should be understood in the total context of social relations, which also includes the life story and the personal mythology of the actual person.

In the following passages I shall limit myself to dealing with the personal mythology displayed in psychopathy. Thus we can pose the question of understanding the meaning of psychopathy. I would like to put the question in the following way: What are the possible elements of what we might call the "psychopathic structure?"

Although Freudian psychoanalysis does not talk about psychopathy it pays much attention to and gives a painstaking description of a similar structure: perversion. If one reads the Freudian thinking about perversion and tries to avoid thinking of perverted persons as simple variants (fetishists, voyeurists, exhibitionists etc.) of the given object, one will find a description of a "perverse" structure, which differs from the psychotic and from the neurotic structures in exactly the same way as does the "psychopathic" structure.

It is an important question why Freud was so interested in perversion but did not engage himself in the problem of psychopathy, which is far more important. After all, perverted persons, viewed as developed individualities whose sexuality is compulsive and centered almost exclusively around perverse acts, amount to a relatively small group of people. To me an important part of the answer is that he discovered that we are all perverts under the skin (where the pervert-polymorphous childish part of ourselves is hidden). In the overtly perverted person he found an outspoken expression of the "perverse" structure, which was his real target of study. In fact, in one of his last important papers, "The Splitting of the Ego," he used the concept of fetishism to open up for an even deeper insight into the formation of the ego, that which threatens to wipe out the very concept of ego, which he himself had used until that moment. In the core of Freudian psychoanalysis we find the description of the sexualized power structures and power struggles that take place in the drama of the person — at the entrance from a two-dimensional universe of phantasms into the three-dimensional world of reality mediated by language. Through his language Freud demonstrated that he was also a prisoner of the individual-centered language. At least we are used to reading his text in that way: through the unavoidable "splitting" of the ego we are on the one hand gaining a membership in society, while on the other hand we are suffering an incurable loss of the paradise of the two-dimensional universe. This incurable loss of paradise is documented and displayed in our belief in and our lifelong search for a "true inner self," in our idea about an absolute justice and in our non-historical scientific thinking about given objects. In fact, it seems to be the story about original sin. But is it necessary to look upon the original sin as a sad happening? I regard the original sin as a gift to mankind. From living according to his needs man began working in order to change his world.

With this criticism in mind we can allow ourselves to proceed in the study of the "psychopathic" or "perverse" structure. In general when we speak of and think about perversion we concentrate on the very sexual act, which however is at root nothing but an act that is extraordinarily eroticized.

If we look away from the colorful stamp of eroticism, what are then the characteristics of the pervert and his act?: (a) The act is fundamentally compulsive and leaves no choice for the actor; (b) The actor seems to be compelled to carry into immediate action most of what he imagines, his fantasy life is impoverished, and he has little freedom whether in act or in fantasy; (c) The object of the act has a magical function and fulfills a restricted and rigidly controlled role; and (d) The magical acts are an essential and relatively consistent part of the actor's psychic stability.

This description allows us to put an identity sign between the "psychopathic" and the "perverse" structure, bearing in mind that we have ignored the eroticizing stamps of perversion. In many case histories we can show the insoluble intimacy of the relations between psychopathic and perverse acts. We therefore need no excuse for the identity sign because of our interest in depicting the common structure.

Henry is now 36 years old. He was raised in an ordinary working family. The mother was a housewife. He has an older brother, who is a moralistic bank manager, actively engaged in religious work. The father is described as a reliable and skilled worker and the mother as a gentle and lenient woman, but somewhat dotty and inclined to religious pondering.

During all his schoolyears Henry was very restless and played truant. He had to change school several times. When one was alone with him, he was good, nice and polite. But if one turned one's back on him he was extremely troublesome. He was not lazy but had difficulties in concentration. The main problem with Henry was his bad relationships with his schoolfellows and playmates amongst whom he was not popular. He was dominating, manipulative and very tyrannical towards his younger schoolfellows.

When he left school he chose his own apprenticeship, but stopped after half a year. Since then he has been employed as a common laborer and for a period of time as a sailor, until three years ago when he received a disability pension. He has always been willing to work and in most places he has been described as skilled and reliable. But he did not get on well with his mates and one had to occupy him in a relatively independent role. His work relations have all been of short duration. Quite often he himself stopped the work relationship for no apparent reason. He then often started a drinking bout lasting several days.

Henry had once been married for five years. He had two children in the marriage, but he never engaged himself in the slightest way in the upbringing of the children, although he was gentle and kind to them in a non-engaged way. Since the divorce he has never seen his former wife or the children and has never expressed a feeling of missing them. His wife has described him as good-natured, and indulgent as long as he was sober. However, when he was drunk he was odious and disgusting, revelling in perverse and violent fantasies and practices. On such occasions he frequently beat her up.

Shortly after his release from school Henry was involved in criminality and was taken into custody at various juvenile institutions. Since then he has had a continuing series of imprisonments, although in most instances he served short-term sentences. The institutions and prisons have unanimously described him as good-natured, giddy and silly, shallow and manipulative. Quite often he is caught in petty cheating. Confronted by his superiors he is as a rule very polite, but leaves the impression of paying lip service. In a steadfast, confident setting, however, it is possible to achieve a relative stability in his behavior. In spite of this he may appear confused, despairing and depressed. It is worth noting that he does not get on well with his fellow inmates.

Most of his criminality consists of crime "committed for the sake of gain," which he does not commit in a state of drunkenness or out of poverty or want, but which happens as a consequence of sudden, impulsive instigation or as an outlet for a state of excitement. He himself says that he experiences his criminal acts as a craving for excitement, but he confesses spontaneously that he does not really understand his own acts. Besides his "economic" crimes he has been convicted of acts of violence, sexual immorality and once of rape. His violent acts and his sexual offences are marked with sadism.

Sometimes Henry appears as mentally sick, appealing for help, worried and concerned about the future and his own capacities for "making it." During such periods he complains of visions and fables of a violent and sadistic sexual nature, that force themselves upon his thinking to such a degree that he is overwhelmed by these fantasies. During his more peaceful periods he resists giving shelter to such fantasies. He will then, completely unworried, explain to you that his goal in life is as regularly as possible to achieve a "pleasant ecstasy." His plan for the future is to live with a tranquil woman in a neat house with the predictable status symbols and "have a nice time."

It is striking that he can tell very little concrete about his childhood and his parents; as well his marriage remains vague and unprecise in his descriptions. His father figure is described as an honest man of high moral standards, but very strict in his discipline and demands. During his mentally bad periods, however, he explains in a dramatic fashion how he was regularly beaten up in a cruel way by his father. He perceives his mother as lenient, but with respect to his parents' divorce, strongly suggests that she might have been of easy virtue.

During his "good" and more stable periods Henry several times decided to change his life style in order to meet the moral demands placed upon him. As an immediate consequence he adopted a new name. He is aware that he did not become another person through this change of name, but ascribes a certain magical power to the change of name that may be of help in solidifying his decision about living a normal life. On the whole it is almost pathetic to observe the hectic persistence he may show in his work at being a normal and reliable citizen. Often he will come in a straightforward way to his superior (or his therapist) to present his "role" as a new man, asking for confirmation and praise of his work. However, if one has to say no to one of his wishes, one may then observe how "loose" and superficial this "role" is. In a prison he is able to handle the situation and keep on with his "role" work.

The psychopathic or perverse structure has to be read as a drama, a stage performance, which at the same time is a defiant challenge to and a denial of the father and thereby of the society as a whole, and a repeated attempt at regaining this lost inner object. The father figure is represented externally from the phallic imago, the third dimension. In order to fully understand the drama of the psychopathic structure we must incorporate the whole setting, which also includes the audience. The anonymous spectator represents the phallic imago, the law, the third dimension. The presence of the spectator and his eventual sentence is decisive to the continuation of the game. For the psychopathic actor the presence of the shadowy third person is a necessity and a constant threat giving rise to a hopeless feeling of depressive guilt. The only way the actor finds to avoid the feeling of depressive guilt is to continue to create acts of illusions, "as if" games through which he defies all rules in deceiving and humiliating the phallic imago. This line of thinking also enables us to conceive of the function and the meaning of the prison institution as "The Theatre of Guilt."

Psychopathy is a drama about a peculiar solution to the oedipal conflict, in which we find a negative mirroring of the "splitting of the ego." The parental imagos are reversed in the way that the father is represented as a cipher of no use as a model for identification, and the mother idealized and endowed with the phallic imago, which however is unattainable because of the presence of reality expressed through the language of the third dimension, the law. If the idealized mother in the interests of reality has produced resistance to the "wishes," she may turn into a deceitful whore. These are the outspoken family portraits; in the unconscious we find a dangerously omnipotent mother threatening to swallow and destroy the child, and an idealized father, a fantasy of an idealized phallus. This ever-present demand for an idealized phallus helps to explain the compulsive character of the psychopathic structure, since its function is to intervene between the child and the dangerous mother. In the internal world of the psychopathic actor the idealized phallus is missing. Instead it is looked for in an external object or situation. The missing idealized phallus is precisely the defect of character that we are usually talking about when describing the psychopath.

The psychopathic structure may be considered as a frozen moment between the anxiety of the psychosis and the depressive guilt of the neurosis, and as an actual non-solution to the oedipal conflict. Being at the same time a bulwark against psychosis and a defense against the depressive guilt, it has to be repeated again and again in acts, that have the character of a play, a game, the meaning of which is forgotten or lost for the actor.

Of course there are differences between psychopathy and perversion, and these should not be neglected, but the basic structure of the two seems to me to be identical, converging at the point of the missing idealized phallus, which in turn may be considered due to a failure in symbolization.

In my treatment of perversion I have drawn heavily on the brilliant paper of Joyce McDougall on the perverse structure.[4] She states several times that many cases of addiction, of delinquency, and of severe "acting out" character pathology, show similar mental mechanisms as those seen in perversion. Furthermore, I fully agree with her when she says that this structure offers an important field of research into the problem of human identity. The idealized phallus, which shows itself so dominantly in all its importance, exactly through its absence in the compulsion of psychopathic acting, may be of great help in understanding how the objective social results of behavior return to the individual in the form of psychological results.

The primary mechanism operating in the psychopathic structure is disavowal (Verleugnung), denial of reality in word and act, which as pointed out by McDougall, implies the notion of avowal (an open confession of knowledge and deed) followed by a destruction of meaning, disavowal. Using the terminology

---

[4] Joyce McDougall, "Primal Scene and Sexual Perversion," *Int. Journal Psycho-Anal.* 53 (1972): 371–384.

of the French psychoanalyst, Jacques Lacan, one might say, that the "pene-trance" of the "signifier" into the story (*étage*) of the "signified" is missing or is insufficient in the psychopathic speech. The psychic representatives of the fetish (objects or situations) and the relations between these representatives have been denuded, emptied of significance or meaning. To the extent that the individual is able to use external objects and situations symbolically he may be able to compensate for the damage of the psychic representatives through a magical, symbolical play; if not, he is condemned to a psychotic solution.

We may now be able to follow Lucien Sève in his sketching of a scientific theory of personality, which he defines as "a science of the acts of human in-dividuals and consequently a science of the ensemble of acts," carried out in time by these individuals; in other words it is a science of human biography.[5] He advocates an elaboration of "the general theory of the concrete individual and no longer the theory of the general forms of human individuality." A psy-chology of personality assimilating the epistemology of historical materialism may enable us to study a concrete personality scientifically through a concrete study of his characteristic processes of activity and of the concrete dialectic of their relations. Sève suggests, that "if one begins with the concept of the social relations between acts (relations supported by mental relations between behav-ior patterns but which differ from them fundamentally) then it is possible to understand the real nature of the infrastructure of personality," and from there to go on understanding the relations of the whole complex of activities, the superstuctures "and, perhaps, the general laws of development."

What I have said so far may be viewed as a modest, sketchy attempt to fol-low some of these guidelines, an attempt made by a practitioner very eager to understand what is going on in his daily life. I hope I am to be forgiven for the following provisional conclusion: We are such stuff that dreams are made of, and our little life is surrounded by history.

[5] Lucien Sève, *Marxism and the Theory of Human Personality* (London: Lawrence and Wishart, 1975).

Comments on Jensen's "The Mask of Psychopathy"

Commentator: A. M. Roosenburg

Dr. Jensen has discussed the words *psychopath* and *psychopathy,* and I wish to comment on his reflections. I think it is of the utmost importance to reflect carefully on words we use, especially on words which so influence our interactions with our fellow men.

Dr. Jensen states that the psychopath is a fiction as the normal man is a fiction. That the last is true, all of us have experienced in life. We all have met people who look "just normal." There seems to be nothing special about them until we get to know them better. Then their individual qualities, hopes, and fears begin to show — and also their peculiarities. The words "just normal" don't fit anymore and it becomes clear that they mean only that the behavior of the "just normal" person will be rather predictable if you meet him superficially. The same is true of the psychopath. The word *psychopath* evokes the expectation of disagreeable behavior in superficial meeting and also the expectation that more than superficial meeting will be difficult. But in getting to know a person labeled as a psychopath, it becomes clear that this is an individual with his own personal qualities, longings and despairs.

It may be clear that we wrong a person when we put him in a category of "normal person," or of "psychopath." We should realize that we are talking about categories of behavior. In my opinion this is of the utmost importance, for behavior is not static but depends upon reaction. This is what Dr. Jensen means when he says that psychopathy is a dynamic form of communication that implies that treatment or change is possible.

The rationale for the existence of the criminal justice system is to give the community an instrument with which to regulate the behavior of its citizens, so that they can live and develop themselves, respecting life and the development of others. It is relevant to evaluate whether the means used by the system are fit to achieve its goals. For instance, is the penal process, and are the sanctions available to the court, optimal to achieve change in the desired direction in that dynamic form of behavior which we call psychopathy and which expresses itself so often in threatening criminal behavior? It is common knowledge that this seems not to be the case. On the contrary, people working in the field of criminal justice and corrections have a growing conviction that the means, designed to correct criminal behavior, have the unwanted side effect of creating more criminal behavior. On psychopathic behavior especially, the effect has never been favorable. I think all this is not so much astonishing as it is predictable. What is astonishing to me is that the knowledge about development in influencing human behavior, gathered by different scientific disciplines has,

---

*Director Emeritus, Dr. Henri van der Hoeven Clinic, Utrecht, Netherlands.

until now, had nearly no influence on penal procedure and sanctions. The reason for this could be that the first reaction of everyone confronted with something threatening is defense. To me, the penal policy as it functions is defensive, and directed against the *persons* who prove to be criminals. It is not really designed to change their behavior, but more to punish them for what they did. The attention during the penal process is directed toward the past, toward the criminal act that happened, toward the guilt of the offender, and toward retribution. The attention is not directed toward the interaction between offender and victim, not directed toward the question of taking responsibility for the consequences of the criminal act, the question of developing more considerate behavior in the future or the whole question of reconciliation. The same can be said of the sanctions available in penal procedure, especially of involuntary commitment to prison for punishment, but also of the involuntary commitment meant for psychiatric treatment. This last is not only treatment-directed but also punitive and repressive.

It is unrealistic to hope that procedures serving conflicting goals will work out satisfactorily in any one direction. If the concern about the ineffectiveness of crime prevention by the penal procedure is serious, the first thing necessary is to set clear goals and choose between the moralizing and the socializing model and then to create a procedure which achieves the chosen goal so that everybody involved works in the chosen direction. Only if the goal is clear will it be possible to evaluate through research whether the means used to achieve the goal are effective and if not, how they could be made more effective.

I know that I risk the reproach of not taking seriously the danger of criminal behavior, but I am convinced that the reproach is unjust. I have worked since 1949 in forensic psychiatry and since 1955 in the treatment of the so-called "dangerous psychopaths." I can assure you that it makes all the difference for the patient if the people emotionally relevant to him (and here I don't only mean his family and those involved in his treatment, but also his judge and his lawyer) expect him to work toward more responsible and less risky behavior.

Comments on Jensen's "The Mask of Psychopathy"

Commentator: Bruno M. Cormier*

In his Introduction to the English translation (1959) of Schneider's book, *Clinical Psychopathology*,[1] Henderson remarks that "his work on psychopathic personality is his most enduring and significant. . . ." He also points out that it is in Schneider's work on psychopathic personality that we find "the greatest divergences from current Anglo-Saxon views" — and, we may add, North American views. It is for this reason that I familiarized myself, to a moderate extent, with Schneider's work. Henderson states that "Schneider's concept of psychopathy stands in direct contrast to the psychoanalytic," namely, to the character neurosis. This contrast is not of great importance, however, if we look at Schneider's work and that of others who have contributed to the knowledge of psychopathy, with a mind that is ready to accept any constructive contribution, taking into account the different frames of reference, schema or theories they represent.

In Schneider's thinking, psychopathy arises from a largely inborn constitution defined as "the totality of the morphological organism with its spontaneous and reaction function. . . ." Referring to constitution, however, he clearly states: "we should not . . . try to equate constitution too narrowly with hereditary endowment. Exogenous intrauterine factors may have influential effect, so, in fact, can the first years of life; these are factors to which the innate disposition is not fundamentally a party . . . constitution is not limited by any metaphysical notion of 'something made once and for all'."[2]

The contrast between Schneider's views and psychoanalytic theory would be very great if the latter theory on the problem of psychopathy or character neurosis had been resolved, as Henderson states, solely "in terms of faulty infantile development — to be treated by psychotherapy or in any case to be explained in purely psychological terms."[3] We must recognize that this psychoanalytic view has found great acceptance in American thinking. In their explanation of Freud's views on psychopathy or psychopathological states, commentators, sometimes psychoanalysts themselves, neglect to stress that Freud always recognized constitutional and hereditary factors, as standing for what we are born with, and also environmental or social factors. Having acknowledged this, he immediately proceeded to construct what became psychoanalysis, centered around human relationships which, from the time of birth on, shape what man

*Professor, Department of Psychiatry and Director, Clinic in Forensic Psychiatry, McGill University, Montreal H2W 1S4, Canada.

[1] Kurt Schneider, *Clinical Psychopathology* (New York: Grune & Stratton, 1959), introduction.

[2] *Ibid.*, p. 16.

[3] *Ibid.*, p. x.

becomes and can explain and possibly undo pathological processes that arise in this epigenetic development. This epigenetic development takes place in a society that has its own historical dialectic evolution.

Another of Schneider's statements on abnormal personality or psychopathic personality (he uses the terms interchangeably) illustrates how far removed Anglo-Saxon, and particularly American, psychiatry's concept of psychopathy and psychopathic personality is from his views. On this subject he states: "abnormal personality implies deviation from some notion we have of average personality. . . . Abnormal personalities merge without any sharp dividing line into what is commonly described as the normal. Among abnormal personalities we distinguish a group of what we call psychopathic personalities. By these we mean people who suffer from their abnormality or whose abnormality makes society suffer. Both types overlap."[4]

I shall not proceed to further discussion of Schneider, but I wanted to illustrate clearly that the terms "psychopathy" and "psychopaths" as they are commonly used in North America and in continental Europe have entirely different meanings. I felt it was important to stress that the approach to the problem of psychopathy, as expounded by Schneider and as implied in Jensen's paper, is not a concept that implies in itself a moral or social judgment, although a capacity to live according to some moral or social rules may be implied. North American use of the term psychopathy is impregnated with moral and social judgment which stems more from a theological morality than from a morality arising from social contracts mentioned by Jensen. This is well illustrated by the fact that it is not uncommon for psychiatrists to say that, faced with a psychopath, they must choose one of two labels, "mad" or "bad."

Some years ago, psychiatrists came to believe that the now abrogated Durham Rule had solved this dilemma. Indeed this statement is partly a caricature, but the fact remains that where the Durham Rule prevailed for some years, many of those who were considered "bad" became legally "mad," even though this did not change the basic problem of psychopathy other than by creating a hospital which had many of the characteristics of a prison. When the Durham Rule is finally assessed, I doubt whether we will be advanced in our knowledge of psychopathy beyond playing games with two labels. However, the Durham Rule may prove to have been somewhat useful if, in the long run, these two labels of "bad" and "mad" disappear altogether from the vocabulary of psychiatry and we start again to question ourselves about the problem of psychopathy. We, as well as the generations to come, should be prepared to revise our views periodically on this topic, since it will take different forms, as Jensen suggests in his dialectic approach to the subject. In that respect I find his paper stimulating. His approach to how the psychopath deals with the problem of morality raises numerous questions with some of which I would now like to deal.

Before proceeding to the discussion of morality and psychopathy, as expounded in Jensen's paper, there is one statement that I would like to have clarified. I would like to be reassured that it does not mean what I read into it. When I see the whole context of the paper, I am confident that I will be reassured, especially as the statement to which I refer follows one which says that

---

[4] *Ibid.*, p. 15.

at times psychiatrists actively "contribute to the confusion around the concept of psychopath" and gives as an example the McCord and McCord view claiming that psychopathy constitutes a threat to the American way of life. The statement to which I am referring is the following: "as psychiatry, besides being a control system of social deviancy, also pretends to be a science, I feel compelled, being a psychiatrist, to try to clarify some important points about the concept of psychopathy."

To what extent psychiatry and its practice is a science or an art is a minor point. The part of the statement that is of much concern to me is that psychiatry is, among other things, a control system of social deviancy. If the statement really means that, then I certainly would strongly object to it. My feelings are quite the opposite: that any deviant (or deviancy) who does not in fact interfere with individual human rights should, in psychiatry, find the strength to be different if he so wishes and some help in coping with the problem of being different. This right, which Nicholas Kittrie refers to as the right to be different, is a most important one, as in a dialectic historical perspective some deviancy has often been the forerunner of the modelling of new values and coming changes. I would certainly begin to worry if psychiatry were to be a control of social deviancy. I obviously give to both expressions, control systems and social deviancy, their broadest meaning, and perhaps Jensen had something more subtle in mind in this paragraph.

Morality and the Law

I am somewhat concerned by the fact that the paper puts so much emphasis on morality and guilt. I feel there is great danger in approaching the problem this way, in that the concept of psychopathy, as conceived in the continental literature, would gradually find its way to becoming an entity filled with moral and social judgments as it is in North America, rather than remaining a clinical entity.

Morality, as defined by Jensen, finds its roots in social contracts and thus has the same roots as the law. I have no quarrel with the notion of morality and law arising from a social contract and of the morality and law of today being the result of a dialectical, historical development. I find it an over-simplification, however, to state that law, and by implication morality, finds its roots only in social contracts. Historically speaking, when we look at morality and law, it is in retrospect that we say they are the result of social contracts. Originally, however, it was men themselves, from the knowledge of their inner world, needs and impulses, who refrained from acting out certain impulses as they realized these were damaging to themselves and to other persons to whom they related. In coming to social contracts to formulate morality and law, men looked at themselves in group relationships, from which emerged new needs or impulses that they found it wiser to be protected against. Thus, both individual and collective psychology are very much at the base of the formulation of laws or rules and morality. As clinicians, we have to deal with reaction, conflict, guilt, fear and anxiety, and once we acknowledge that law and morality should be looked at as different, though having common origins, what we are concerned with is how one deals with law and morality.

In my view, guilt feelings and morality are too central to Jensen's presentation. Although guilt is a form of individual and social control, it is far from being the strongest one. Guilt, for example, may come after the act is committed
rather than before, especially when one realizes that an object of relationship is
lost, and the guilt that exists is really more because of the loss than because of
the destructive act itself. I could give many examples of this where superego,
and guilt arising from superego values, are not as strong controls as they are
sometimes represented to be. I, for example, find a more important source of
control in the capacity to feel depressed about oneself and others, the capacity
to feel regret and concern about oneself and the opinion of others. I am aware
that if one has such an emotional balance that all these functions and others are
present, the capacity to experience guilt is there, but this is precisely the point
that I want to make, namely, that in psychological development, the capacity
to feel comes first. In classical Greece they had two words to express two very
important basic feelings, one of which is still currently used, i.e., "sympathy,"
to suffer with, expressly to suffer with somebody or share the suffering of
somebody. There was also another word which has been lost, "symphyly,"
which is the counterpart of the first, "to love with." In other words, relationships involve these two capacities, to be able to share the suffering that another
person undergoes, and to be with one who suffers, but also to be pleased that
somebody is loved, and to share and love in that way and in doing so to share
and love with others — the exact counterpart of sympathy. The capacity to feel
is, in our view, a most important development in human beings and it is an impairment in this development that is at the center of psychopathy rather than
the incapacity to experience guilt. This latter point will be the object of our
conclusions.

To return to the social contracts that give rise to morality and law, Jensen's
paper presents further complications, beginning with the question of what is
covered by morality and law? In my view, morality and law sometimes cover
quite different territories, although both emerge from social contracts. Although they cover the same ground in many areas, there are many things which
are frowned upon by moral values which are by no means against the law, nor
should they be. Indeed, the contrary statement could be made for laws regarding morality. Thus, in many ways, if one associates psychopathy with morality,
as Jensen and some others do, and with an inability to comply with the rules
dictated by law, one finds oneself in a curious sort of situation of ultimately
having to make up one's mind about which moral rules or laws, not accompanied by guilt feelings, will decide that you are suffering from psychopathy. I
find this situation rather uncomfortable.

In thinking of present-day morality, some of us are not ready to feel guilty
about many precepts of contemporary morality and in a number of areas of
morality one is left to one's own judgment and conscience. Compared to the
concept of guilt based on introjected values, i.e., superego, what I have referred
to in a previous paper as "ego morality" may well be a more important form of
control in individual and social relationships. While I will not elaborate on this
concept of ego morality at this stage, suffice it to say that it is well expressed in
daily life by the idea of what the neighbors might think, or what one would

think of oneself in the commission of certain acts. In other words, what others feel about "me" and how I feel about myself are strong ego feelings in human relationships.

Guilt and the Concept of Responsibility

After having made these remarks on the role of the superego in the control of social conduct, I had a personal talk with Dr. Roosenberg about her statement that the important thing in the treatment of those whom we call or who are labelled "psychopaths" is that they reach the point where they accept responsibility for their acts. My understanding is that this acceptance of responsibility does not necessarily imply that the person really grasps and accepts all the implications and consequences for himself and others, including regret, remorse, and so on, but that they have reached the point of accepting that they are the perpetrators of the acts they have committed, without exaggerating or minimizing their deeds either to save face or for secondary gain.

An acceptance of that reality, even if it is not accompanied by anxiety, concern, or regret, is a real achievement in the treatment of those who have been called psychopaths. Often, it may appear that they recognize that they are the author of the deeds of which they have been found guilty, but those who work with them know how many mechanisms are used to deny responsibility for their acts. In their language they have been "framed," been unlucky, somebody else made a mistake, and the means whereby they tend to maximize or minimize their involvement, as mentioned above is another way of modifying their recognition that what they have committed is real; this needs to be established if a dialogue is to take place about the deed and its author. If Dr. Roosenberg's concept of responsibility implies a practical recognition of the fact that the man is the author of an act for which he may not otherwise feel anxiety, affect or guilt, this acceptance that he is the author, without rationalization or distortion, is a necessary testing of reality that is the beginning that allows him to go beyond the act to find the hidden motivation and affects. Such a down-to-earth approach to a concept of responsibility is essential in the approach to the people we call psychopaths but whom I personally prefer to describe within the frame of a nosography of personality or character disorder.

The Problem of Psychopathy

It is not possible for us to work with a clinical concept, referred to as a syndrome or diagnosis, basically characterized by antisocial behavior and an absence of guilt vis-à-vis such behavior. To refer to some persistent offenders as psychopaths or as suffering from psychopathy is not clinically useful. It is against medical or psychiatric thinking not to look at a problem in all its dimensions in a man that is taken as a whole. While acknowledging and, as a psychiatrist, using the great contributions made by sociologists and criminologists in criminal and anti-social behavior, I deplore that too many psychiatrists have accepted that a form of behavior that we do not like becomes a symptom and sometimes the only symptom that is looked at. For me, such an attitude indicates an important area of psychiatric blindness in looking at anti-social behavior in all its dimensions. Having worked for so many years now with persistent offenders, in and out of prison, I am obliged to admit that I never saw any who correspond to the too-precise description that so-called "psychopaths" have been given since as far back as Pinel and Pritchard. I feel rather more comfortable studying those who, among other things, repeatedly committed anti-social acts and presented many other symptoms in affect, thinking and behavior, symptoms that are as severe as their anti-social acts, and sometimes more so. While I understand that society must, for the welfare of the citizens of the state, deal with behavior that it cannot condone, I do not, as a clinician, feel that my clinical judgment should be influenced by protection of the citizen or society. Fortunately, other professionals are well trained to do that. As a psychiatrist I feel that I should be as objective as I can in studying any man whom I have accepted to assess or treat. I deplore the fact that psychiatrists, who are basically doctors and most of the time fairly objective in studying diagnosis or behavior that basically implies moral and social judgment, react to this behavior as badly as the ordinary citizen and sometimes worse. There is unfortunately a lot of truth in what a well-known penitentiary commissioner told a psychiatric meeting of which he was the guest — that he found as much prejudice in psychiatrists as in other classes of citizens. One of our contentions is that the great importance placed on superego in persistent offenders is an aspect of these prejudices rather than a clinical finding.

I am aware, however, that in making these criticisms one is not contributing much to the solution of the problem and for that reason I would like to conclude by offering some of the ideas and concepts that have guided our work with persistent offenders — those we call anti-social — during nearly a quarter of a century, and would like to sum up these principles in a few brief statements.

1. We believe that persons who show anti-social behavior, among other findings, should find their place within the classification of character neurosis and we should not establish a special diagnosis to account for this behavior. When Henderson refers to psychopathic states and describes the many entities in which they can be found, his approach does not involve social and moral judgment but an honest and objective approach, now considered as a classic in psychiatry, to understand states that, among other things, involve unacceptable behavior.[5] Schneider's approach, already mentioned, is another one that excludes moral judgment.

2. If we are to understand character neurosis or any syndromes in ego formation that lead to social pathology, we must also accept what appears to us evident that ego formation and development do not stop at a certain state but undergo changes that involve complex processes from the early formative years up to death. These changes had been most observed in those referred to as psychopaths, persistent offenders, or hard-core criminals. If one wants to place them in a definite syndrome or diagnosis, one must at least recognize that those who are referred to as sociopaths or other labels change dramatically as they pass through the different cycles of life and this must make us less secure in label-

⁵ D. K. Henderson, *Psychopathic States* (London: Chapman & Hall, 1939).

ling them with ill-defined diagnoses that unfortunately too often involve the moral and social judgment already mentioned and lead to a nihilistic approach to their understanding and to their treatment. Even if the treatment consists of not much more than an attentive observation of how they evolve, and a serious attempt to explain how, in their late 30s and early 40s, those we have called psychopaths no longer justify this label, this type of unbiased approach will ultimately bear fruit.

3. Our last remark will deal with psychopathology and what we consider an important nucleus of those who display a long history of acting out that interferes with harmonious relationships in individual and social life. This concluding remark is taken from a paper written with a colleague, Dr. S. Simons.[6]

Psychiatrists who deal with persistent criminals have always had and continue to have difficulty in understanding them, particularly in experiencing enough empathy to establish a therapeutic relationship. No matter how well they can describe the many personality disturbances encountered, they remain baffled by the persistent, repetitive, anti-social acting out, and perhaps even more by the relative equanimity with which these men accept retaliation in the form of punishment, often harsh, and often leading to a waste of many years in their lives.

Acting out is pathology of action, and persistent delinquency is most certainly a serious form of chronic pathological action. Action, whether pathological or normal, is an ego function, as is thought and affect. In structural terms, although this is an over-simplification, we can distinguish an action ego, a thought ego and an affect ego. Action, thought, and affect comprise the total of behavior, and normality can be seen as a harmonious balance and co-operation within these three ego substructures. These substructures of the ego derive energy from the instinctual drives, and the quantitative distribution of drive energy that is taken up by each of these substructures is important, as is their capacity to handle and transform this energy. In delinquency, the action ego is hypercathected and its function pathological. In contrast, thought and affect are hypocathected. It is true that the description of delinquents as deficient in thought and affect is in many ways correct; they do not think ahead nor learn from past experience, and their affect is shallow. This does not imply that the capacity is in itself lacking or that this remains so.

We find it useful to treat the persistent offender as a person within this theoretical frame of reference, i.e., a man who hypercathected action to the extent that in his early development he could not pass to the subsequent necessary phase, where acting gradually becomes attached to affect so that to act and to feel gradually become inter-related, and at the same time balances and controls become established. In a third phase, thinking — words being the ultimate expression of thinking — is added to form the core of what we are, namely, human beings who act, feel and think. Some historians hold that first came the dance (movement, or the act), then poetry (the affect), followed by the word (thinking or philosophy). Persistent delinquents take a long time to achieve this evolution and to synthesize this trilogy, but in the end they come to some sort

---

[6] Siebert P. Simons and Bruno M. Cormier, "Delinquent Acting Out and Ego Structure," *Laval Médical* 40 (November 1969): 932–935.

of solution as shown by the abatement of criminality with the process of aging. It is when they reach adulthood, sometime in their 30's, that most persistent offenders (whom so many psychiatrists refer to as psychopaths) come to the conclusion that some way, somehow, sometime in their life, reason or thinking must prevail.

On this long way to realizing that thought or reason must prevail, the persistent offender goes through many conflicts which are well known in classical literature. In the opening passages of Goethe's *Faust*, we see our hero with all the wisdom of the world, dissatisfied and weary, pondering over the meaning of the mysterious opening words of the Gospel of St. John, "En archei eh ho logos," — "In the beginning was the Word." He considers the traditional translation, considers the alternatives of logos, such as idea or thought, and rejects them all. The correct meaning, he decides, should be, "In the beginning was the deed," and, having concluded his pact with the devil, he acts, in fact he acts out. A hundred years later, Freud, in his essay, *Totem and Taboo,* traces the beginnings of morality, ethics, and social cohesion, man's propensity to neurosis, to the original crime, the murder of the father. He speculates at the end of the essay whether this original crime took place in reality, and favors this assumption by quoting Goethe's words, "In the beginning there was the deed."

For our delinquent patients, one might say this is true also; for them in the beginning was the deed, but they are not hypothetical, primitive man at the threshold of true human experience. They can postpone, but in the end they do not escape the human condition. For them, too, eventually logos, instead of deed, becomes word, or idea, or emotion, or command, if you like.

If we have left out consideration of the superego, we are aware of an omission and an over-simplification, and can, therefore, in this brief statement, do no better than refer to the subsequent words of the Evangelist, who knew this all along. "And the word was God," which, interpreted non-theologically, represents values, conscience and superego.

The Many-Headed Psychiatrist

Michael Zeegers*

In ancient times, and even now among some isolated tribes, the medicine man was and is a holy man, a mystic being, sometimes venerated and treated with the respect due a god. In Homer's Iliad[1] we read that one single doctor is worth a multitude of ordinary people. This statement still holds true — the doctor is not an ordinary being; a magician of sorts, he guards us from danger lurking in every corner, defends us, and is above all a warrior.

The psychiatrist, likewise a physician, bears traits of a god, a priest, a king, or indeed a heroic warrior. Alas, recently even the psychiatrist is a contested character. He may sometimes be looked upon with apprehension. There are some who consider him a menace, a disease producing pathogenic factor, a hindrance to progress and recovery. Scrutinized, he has his antagonists — sometimes psychiatrists themselves — called anti-psychiatrists.

Sketching a vignette of man or woman whose task it is to keep a watch over people's mental health is a sheer impossibility. But we might find refuge in mythology, where we read of a many-headed being, the Hydra. That image serves our purpose. The actual description of a Hydra according to Webster's dictionary reads: "A many-sided problem or obstacle that presents new difficulties each time one aspect of it is solved or overcome." We might contemplate the nature of the heads this creature possesses.

The Head of a Physician

The psychiatrist is a physician to begin with, and as such he partakes of the glory of a lengthy line of respectable doctors, and of the tribute paid to them. The doctor Aesculapius was adored in ancient Greece. The famous Dutch humanist Erasmus, once wrote an *Encomium Artis Medicae,*[2] a praise of the art of medicine. "We owe much gratitude," Erasmus said, "to the physician, who engages himself in a continual struggle against the many enemies of our lives." He esteemed him above a king — for a king may spare a man's life by not putting him to death; a doctor, however, actually snatches him out of the very jaws of death. We must also bear in mind that Erasmus wrote his *Encomium Moriae,*[3] The Praise of Folly, which rendered him immortal. This fact might cause us to become suspicious. Should we not distrust his sincerity, when his abundant praise of medicine is almost embarassing? Yet we know that his *En-*

---

*Professor of Forensic Psychiatry, Leyden University, Holland.
[1]Homer, *Iliad* (book XI, 514).

[2]Desiderius Erasmus, *Encomium Artis Medicae* (original 1518).

[3]Desiderius Erasmus, *Encomium Moriae* (original 1511) *The Praise of Folly*, (Ann Arbor: The University of Michigan Press, 1958).

comium Moriae was no mere joke. In this work we encounter irony, satirical criticism, skepticism, but also recognize sincerity, earnestness and paradoxes revealing wisdom of the highest order.

We may therefore allow the psychiatrist to wear the trappings of a physician with pride. Medical research in the psychiatric field, in combination with diagnosis and treatment, has indeed borne fruit. It is true that medical thinking has its limitations. A one-sided viewpoint may even be dangerous. In studying deviant behavior the physician may show a tendency to classify any deviance as an illness. He may employ his medicinal armament, i.e., prescriptions, or even surgical treatment for abnormal behavior, too readily. He may, by focusing all his attention upon the patient, lose sight of the pathogenic factors in the latter's family and in society. It is important to admit that these limitations are real, that these dangers exist, and to acknowledge also that errors are being made. Nosological classification in psychiatry has been far from successful, and hospital treatment sometimes induces pathological symptoms, rather than reducing them. Social problems are often overlooked. This blind spot may reach pathological dimensions, and here and there psychiatrists are being misused and are exploiting their positions for the sake of social and political control. Let us take the words "here and there" literally: It not only happens there; it may also refer to us, here, as well.

All the same I do not advocate that we behead the doctor. Medical education sharpens our vision, medical examination teaches us to look at the various contributing factors of the case, and medical diagnosis, if properly used, provides us with real gnosis – insight. I would like to emphasize that these particular medical terms are being employed here for good reason. The medical man knows that symptoms have a particular significance in diagnosis, such as those encountered with an inflammation. They not only indicate the presence of illness, but are also an expression of the body's reaction against the noxae which caused them. E.g., fever reaction is one of the defensive reactions – a weapon the patient requires in order to survive.

This also applies to neurotic or psychotic symptoms, as they too have a significance, and are not only a signal of distress. These symptoms indicate to us the manner in which the patient is struggling. In the same way that his body may require fever in the combating of toxins he may also require his depressive reaction, his delusion, and neurotic mechanisms as a defense against overwhelming forces. We can only be of help to him if we learn to recognize and understand the language of these symptoms.

In this context Hughlins Jackson's views are deserving of mention, which have been more amply discussed in Hans Oppenheimer's interesting book *Clinical Psychiatry*.[4] Of special interest is the distinction Jackson made between positive and negative symptoms, which can be applied to psychiatry as well as neurology. For example a paralysis is a negative symptom which may be due to a lesion of the brain. A tremor is a positive symptom which can never be the product of a lesion, but can only be produced by intact areas; their pathological activity is related to the lesion, but in fact finds its origin in other parts of the brain. A delusion or hallucination is not the product of a toxic agent, nor of

---

[4]Hans Oppenheimer, *Clinical Psychiatry: Issues and Challenges* (New York: Harper & Row, 1971).

a brain lesion, but is instead the product of a man whose reactions are the very expression of his need and struggle. This also holds true for some criminal acts committed by disturbed people. When an aged man suffering from arteriosclerotic dementia commits a sexual assault upon a child, his act and his sexual desire are not the products of his arteriosclerotic vessels, nor of his damaged brain cells. Of course his acts, his movements and his feelings are connected with brain cells that are still unimpaired. We used to solve our problem by saying that he had lost control. It seems more exact to conclude that this man stands in life in an altered way, as a result of his deficiency. His psychic and his physical achievements are impaired. He is often aware of his shortcomings, which hamper his social possibilities and make him suffer. He feels inferior and isolated. We will never be able to indicate an exact spot in the brain from which the crime arises. But we can say that it is the unimpaired part of his personality that reacts to his situation — having to live with his deficiencies. We may conclude that medical research has made a considerable contribution to our insight, and to our knowledge of man; in daily practice the psychiatrist remains a solace and a comfort for many people.

The Head of a King

In earlier times the doctor displayed the salient characteristics of an absolute monarch. However, in the present day this type of doctor has been dethroned. He is no longer the sole master of diagnosis and treatment, and works in cooperation with biochemists, physicists and sociologists. He consults with statisticians, economists and planning experts, and is often the teammate of psychologists and social workers. In such company it would seem unfitting to appear garbed in the raiments of royalty. Thus the physician is drawn closer to ordinary people, a decided advantage for him and them.

The Head of a Poker Player

A few years ago Verhulst, a Belgian psychiatrist, published a book in which he described the practice of medicine as being like a game of poker.[5] Psychiatry is regarded as entirely dependent upon chance, not only with respect to the type of treatment a patient receives but even with regard to the kind of illness that may develop. The odds are determined by the decisions made by the doctor, his views and methods. Of course in the case of a broken leg, the surgeon's skill, in conjunction with his devotion and attitude are of paramount importance; in psychiatry however there is a more essential issue at stake. The question, "What does the doctor make of it?" often has a literal meaning. The doctor makes his diagnosis, and in so doing he marks the client out for illness. His diagnosis has a stigmatizing effect, with the result that the doctor may become a pathogenic factor. When a young man refuses to accept the standards of his parents, uses drugs, or is a conscientious objector, the psychiatrist is approached for advice and counsel. What does he make of it? He may inform the perturbed

---

[5] Johan Verhulst, *Pokerspel geneeskunde* [Medicine, a poker-game], (Antwerpen-Utrecht: De Nederlandsche boekhandel, 1972).

parents that their son is expressing his independence as a free citizen, and that his disobedience and adventurous spirit are just the attitudes we need in the land of the free and the home of the brave. The psychiatrist may also react to this situation by making predictions of mental illness and a criminal career as an unavoidable consequence. Should the young man in question not pay heed, the psychiatrist could only classify him as belonging to the genus: personality disorders. Another psychiatrist might commence upon an analysis of the patient's childhood, impulses and instincts — and he in turn will be disposed to label him as neurotic or even possibly schizophrenic. These different diagnostic labels are not free of danger, as that which we call a rose by any other name would smell as sweet; but that which we call a common rebel will not develop in the same way by any other name; say by the name of a psychopath, a neurotic or a schizophrenic, or simply a patient.

Our medical diagnosis also includes a prediction, and this prediction may produce effects of its own. The astronomer when predicting an eclipse of the moon, does not govern the course of events in the least — however a doctor who predicts mental deterioration does effect the future deportment of his patient. His prophecy is very apt to fulfill itself. So the psychiatrist could be a dangerous man — even if only through his diagnosis. To quote a famous English poet: "A label of illness is a risk forever." When a doctor gets the opportunity to treat the so-called "patient" according to his own views, the riskiness increases: it will never pass into nothingness.

It will be clear that in forensic psychiatry these risks increase all the more. The psychiatrist's report is sometimes decisive in criminal cases, and is often the last word when disability is judged in social legislation. I have drawn a comparison between medical prognosis and astronomical prediction. Alas, not only do the doctor's prophecies bear more consequences as to the future course of events, but they are also much less exact, and of limited objectivity. Doctors often disagree amongst themselves concerning psychiatry; yet they present their opinions as facts — with a distinct air of self-confidence and authority.

The Head of a Priest

The introduction of this topic ushers us back to the very dawn of medicine and human knowledge. Ancient mythological thinking was based on the assumption that all events were principally determined by Divine intervention. So far as we know, logical causality was introduced into our Western culture by Thales of Milet around 600 B.C. Between 800 and 200 B.C. we find in China, India, Iran, Palestine, and Greece, in remarkable synchronism, the rise of modern thought. In medical science, Hippocrates of Kos is called the father of modern medicine.

Scientific thinking has never completely superseded the tangled web of mythological thought. Hippocrates never entirely defeated Aesculapius. Demonological thoughts are to be found repeatedly — even in western medical science. This brings to mind Paracelsus, the fifteenth-century physician and chemist, who wrote mystical treatises concerning illness. The first author to have drawn up a classification of mental diseases was Felix Platter (1563—1614), and although he centered his attention upon the physical aspects, he also expressed his opinion that disturbances of the mind were influenced by supernatural powers. A most interesting occurence took place in the year 1775 in Wurtemberg. A renowned religious healer named Johann Joseph Gassner appeared to be experiencing a great deal of success, although his clerical superiors seemed less than enchanted about his activities. The thoughts concerning Enlightenment were in definite discord with those of exorcism. Gassner was later to be out-done by still another miracle healer, one Franz Anton Messmer, who was to be renowned for his so-called magnetism. Messmer, in the presence of experts, demonstrated his ability to provoke similar symptoms to Gassner's — what's more to dispel them without the use of faith healing or exorcism! We could regard Messmer as a pioneer of psychotherapy, although personally he ascribed his successes to the presence of "Magnetism." Unfortunately his theories were disproved during his lifetime. Messmer was an example, though, of successful healers whose results foster erronous theoretical constructions, which are themselves based upon questionable suppositions. Even in our time there exist healers such as Messmer and Gassner.

Rational scientific and religious viewpoints need not contradict one another. The history of psychiatry points us to an example of this in Johann Christian Heinroth (1773–1843). Most people only remember him for his concept that mental illness is the result of sin. This conception appears too simple, or irrational to be noteworthy. Heinroth was however one of the leading psychiatrists of his day, and was the first German professor in the field of psychic medicine, and a foremost clinician. He was in addition the first to use the term 'psychosomatic.' He recommended various psychotherapeutic as well as soma-therapeutic methods.

When considering Heinroth's conception of the relationship between sin and mental illness, his writings should be read in the light of the current thinking of his own day. He did not make mention of the patient's particular sins. On the contrary, he maintained that the physician should not meddle in metaphysical and moral affairs. Alexander and Selesnick have stated that it would suffice to replace the term "sins" with that of "guilt feelings" in order to consider Heinroth an actual predecessor of current psychoanalysis.[6] This opinion is also supported by Ellenberger.[7] I do not feel that this obliging attempt to give Heinroth a modern image does him justice. It carries his conception into the realm of psychology. The concepts of soul, mind, and psyche never fall completely together, as was already made clear by Aristotle. Heinroth's views are not in the same category as psychoanalysis; neither should we identify his ideas with the concept of anomia. His doctrine is far removed from the uncritical movements of religious healing.

A relationship may be established with modern thinking, via Romano Guardini. This philosopher poses the question whether the mind can become ill — not the nervous system alone, nor the psychological functions, — but the mind itself as such. He has pointed toward the alarming experiences of our time, the dangers of power, the systematic destruction and annihiliation of the individual,

[6] Franz G. Alexander and Sheldon T. Selesnick, *The History of Psychiatry* (New York: Harper & Row, 1966).

[7] Henri F. Ellenberger, *The Discovery of the Unconscious* (New York: Basic Books, 1970).

and human rights and values. In analyzing Plato and St. Augustine, he has argued that the mind becomes affected when the relationship with truth, righteousness, and holiness are essentially disturbed. In that case medical therapy can offer no relief; therefore a mental reversal or metanoia would be required, says Guardini.[8] These observations lead us far beyond the realm of psychiatric science; yet we are dealing with very real human problems and with everyday existence. The psychiatrist comes face to face with people who have been confronted with inhumanity and terror; people who have been dealing with evil itself.

In my own country there are a great many people who can never really be liberated after the close of World War II; this because there is no remedy for their distress. When we think of the many wars and outbursts of inhumanity that have taken place during recent decades all over the world; our imagination fails us when attempting to estimate the number of victims overcome by these agonizing events. It is my belief that the psychiatrist cannot do without some understanding in these areas, which, although living outside the actual scope of science, still touch upon his thinking and practice. The psychiatrist must confront the full human problem, including its inherent spiritual aspects. The psychiatrist however should not play the role of priest, and certainly must not make attempts at being a magician.

The Head of a Judge

Another official whose gown indicates his dignified function, is the judge. Sometimes it is feared that the forensic psychiatrist might annex the judge's bench. One ought not to be disturbed, for he only offers his advice, but does not make decisions in a court of law. That is the task of the judge, not only because he is the expert relating to judicial questions, but also because he bears the responsibility, as he is the representative of the government. The judge must give consideration to the elucidations of the psychiatrist, alongside other factors, such as general security, crime prevention, etc. The psychiatrist must remain aloof from pronouncing sentence in a criminal trial.

In Holland there is one occasion in which the psychiatrist forms part of the court, and thus officiates as a judge. When a prisoner has completed at least nine months, and two-thirds of his confinement, the Government may grant him probation. Until three years ago the Government's decision was final, but now the prisoner is offered the possibility of appealing to a special court where he can defend his case. This court consists of three lawyers and two consulting experts, who may be psychiatrists, psychologists, or social workers. In these cases where judgment of personality, social possibilities, and prognosis are essential, the non-lawyers contributions are significant.

In the future this special court will also be charged with cases involving so-called psychopaths who have been ordered to be detained during her Majesty's pleasure, to use the English phrase. The existing possibilities for appeal to the judiciary are generally regarded as unsatisfactory. The patient can hardly defend himself in cases where his physician feels it necessary to extend his term. The power of the psychiatrist is exhorbitant, when his arguments are to be

---

[8]Romano Guardini, *Die Macht* (Würzburg: Werkbund Verlag, 1958).

judged by lawyers only. Here too, psychiatric, psychological and sociological viewpoints should be considered indispensable to see justice done.

The Head of a Police Officer

To make a report in a criminal case we first need to establish a means of making real contact. There may be cases in which the person in question is unconscious or severely psychotic. In these cases no real personal contact is possible. However in the great majority of instances there must exist a bond of understanding between the examiner and examinee. Both parties must cooperate. The suspect must first give his consent to be examined — and then only by a doctor. Needless to say meaningful informed consent can only apply to cases where the patient has some reason to trust the examiner. When we present ourselves as psychiatrists, this also implies that we are doctors. This grants us some rights, but also entails special responsibilities.

There may be pathologists whose task is that of serving the police force, thus combating crime, and apprehending criminals. We cannot however, combine the task of a physician (i.e., confidential contact) with that of a detective (tracking a person down). A psychopathologist who behaves like a prosecuter, or who assists the District Attorney in the interrogation of suspects[9] should not rightly be identified as a psychiatrist, which means after all, a doctor.

By the use of forensic psychiatric reports we may run the risk, that the psychiatrist himself may contribute to the controversy by adding fresh material on the question of guilt. I think the correct attitude to be employed by a physician while examining a suspect, should be always to bear in mind that the doctor is a confidential agent. In cases where the suspect denies his guilt, the doctor will seldom be in a position to give a complete report. If he makes the attempt, he should proceed with extreme caution.

Another instance where the psychiatrist must be very careful is the obtaining of information through persons other than the patient himself. We have all encountered loose remarks made by relatives or neighbors, which have been employed in psychiatric reports as hard facts. The psychiatrists involved have made bad policemen. Real policemen would have been more careful and discreet. Before closing this topic, a special warning should be issued. Words such as hysteria, aggravation, neurotic maneuver, resistance, etc., are apt to be turned around by the prosecution, and used as a dangerous weapon against the one they were intended to protect. In reports and documents, these terms are difficult to dispense with, but we must be conscious of the damage which can be wrought by the flippant utilization of terms such as "psychopath." Though far from being a terrorist, I propose we burn off the police officer's head, should it ever make its appearance upon the psychiatric Hydra.

The Head of a Warrior

The physician is not infrequently glorified as being a heroic soldier, fighting for our welfare. Books like *Microbe Hunters, Hunger Fighters, Men Against Death, Fight for Life,* and *The Citadel* are successful novels about heroic doc-

---

[9] J. Paul de River, *The Sexual Criminal,* 2nd ed. (Springfield, Ill.: Thomas, 1956).

tors, whose continued struggles have fascinated millions. The terminology of war is often employed: fighting disease, battling sickness or bacteria. We even speak of our treatment as being a strategy. There are objections however. A suit of armour does not appear to be an appropriate garment for communication, and is somewhat inflexible as well. We must also acknowledge the fact that man who engages himself in battle must be aggressive, the danger being here that the aggression of the doctor could be inadvertently directed towards the patient himself.

Alexander and Selesnick begin *The History of Psychiatry* with the statement: "The mentally ill have always been with us — to be feared, marvelled at, laughed at, pitied, or tortured — but all too seldom cured!" Not only so-called psychopaths, but also neurotics and severely depressed individuals are often treated as if they were wilful criminals, lazybones, frauds, or at least blockheads who ought to know better. We can hardly begin to imagine the extent of the mischief caused by aggressive psychiatrists. Irreparable loss of confidence, blocked communication, impossibility of further treatment and suicide, are the consequences. The psychiatrist easily asserts that he is not to blame, pointing out instead that these failures are the result of the patient's illness, his strong resistance, or the interference of transference with proper treatment. This situation is even more grave when the client does not consult the doctor of his own free choice. People undergoing treatment in hospitals, or consulting social psychiatrists in their bureaucratic offices, or patients being given forensic examinations, represent the stock categories. I have been made aware of patients who have been in hospital and could only compare their experience with a stay in a concentration camp. Some of them suffer from a pathological syndrome, as a result of the torture and humiliation. I have met people who informed me about psychiatrists who began interviews by making malicious remarks, or by grossly insulting their clients; the elementary rules applying to decency and good manners, seemed to go unobserved. Perhaps you doubt these persons' credibility, but the reports written by these psychiatrists often confirm the client's assertions.

In forensic cases we should not forget that we are dealing with handicapped clients, people who are in a most unfavorable predicament. Being the subject of an examination is a humiliating experience. Being suspected of having committed a crime, or being engaged in a conflict about being unable to work, implies a great disadvantage. More so, as the person involved is the opponent of the experts. Even his lawyer is hardly able to criticize medical opinion. When psychiatrists go to war, their opponents are not to be envied.

The head of a warrior does not fit the psychiatrist. Ultimately psychiatric aggression should be seen as having a paradigmatic significance in the study of human aggression, and might be a suitable medium which could be productively used to sort out the origins of aggressive interaction. We might distinguish between three groups of aggression — promoting variables: (a) those concerning the aggressor, (b) those related to the victim, and finally, (c) situation variables. The term "occasional aggression" has been introduced to indicate the significance of the situation in those cases.[10]

---

[10]T. Fris, *Gelegenheids agressie* [Occasional aggression]. (Meppel: Boom, 1972).

Opportunities for aggression are frequently available to the psychiatrist, and weapons are placed in his hands. Disturbed people are sometimes restless, and their behavior may be alarming or dangerous. Consequently coercive measures have been devised in order to protect the patient and his fellowman. Some of these methods of restraint by force are truly ingenious, as psychiatric history attests, yet these methods themselves are called "defensive." Nevertheless, it is not difficult to expose the subtle aggressive tendencies implied.

The use of these methods influences both the wardens and the therapist, and their handiwork makes them calloused. Treatments like ECT and surgical intervention are somewhat aggressive in themselves, and not only influence the patient's behavior, but also those of the therapists, nurses and doctors.[11] Modern psychotropic drugs not only alter behavior, but also the personality.

Even psychotherapy may be a very effective weapon, and might at times come close to brainwashing. In the late fifties William Sargant published *Battle for the Mind,*[12] a physiology of conversion and brainwashing, as he called it. About this same time Meerloo wrote about *The Rape of the Mind.*[13] Two titles about aggression on the mind, revealing to us the alarming possibilities of psychic power, and the transformation of the free human mind into an automatic responding machine. This poses a real threat to mankind. Ends do not always justify the means, especially when our methods need not be approved by others. *Treatment or Torture*[14] is the title of a book, in which the author states that violation of the personality may readily be achieved by the perversion of the very methods designed to foster the growth and autonomy of the individual. Psychiatrists may become aggressive only because the situation offers them the opportunity.

Looking for aggression-provoking variables lying in the victim, we find a second cause for aggressive psychiatric behavior, namely, frustration-aggression, first described by Dollard, et al. Psychiatric patients put us to a great deal of trouble and frustration. Their own aggressive behavior begs for an answer. We often feel incompetent, helpless, and unable to cope with their symptoms. We cannot always understand them and cannot cure them; moreover they confront us with our own problems, with possibilities which threaten to confuse and debilitate the human mind. Psychiatric patients of all kinds behave in annoying, provocative, and offensive manner. In feeling frustrated one may have the tendency to reflect back their aggressive behavior.

The third group of aggression-provoking variables is to be found within the aggressor himself. I have already mentioned the possibility that aggressive tendencies may cause a person to choose medicine as a career. Some choose surgery, while still others find themselves attracted by psychology and psychiatry. One gets the opportunity to meddle with other people's affairs.

Some fear that people consider psychiatry sissified. Therefore we sometimes feel it necessary to display manly behavior at all costs, and to give a show of

[11] D. W. Abase and J. A. Ewing, "Transference and Countertransference in Somatic Therapies," *The Journal of Nervous and Mental Disease* 123 (1956): 32.

[12] William Sargant, *Battle for the Mind* (London: Heinemann, 1967).

[13] Joost A. M. Meerloo, *The Rape of the Mind* (New York: The Universal Library, 1961).

[14] G. Seaborn Jones, *Treatment or Torture* (London: Tavistock Publications, 1968).

boldness, resolute bearing, and above all, not to allow anybody to think of us as being weak, timid or indeed compassionate. This at least holds true for our Western society. Margaret Mead, as a result of her anthropological studies, settled upon the concept that personality differences between men and women are inherently linked to their sex. We are nonetheless conditioned by our society and culture. Masculine characteristics are still considered a trait of which we are expected to be proud.

The reverse has been shown by Fasteau in his book *The Male Machine*.[15] He depicts men in our society, whose craving for status, lust for power and authority, causes them to destroy their fellowmen, leading the world to the verge of disaster, priding themselves about being hard-nosed businessmen, shrewd politicians, insidious, shifty, and underhanded. Men of prominent position, as well as the slumdweller, literally consume one another in their lust for power and material possessions — and from somewhere produce the nerve to boast about their masculinity. Destructive aggression is to be found in every country, in every part of society, in the youth, as well as in government. This aggression is inextricable from sexuality. We know that the exhibitionist displays his sexuality as evidence of his manliness, and that this behavior is inherent in those who are fundamentally unsure of themselves. There exists also some expression of hostility in their desire to frighten and shock members of the opposite sex. The most important motivating factor is the need for reassurance.

The psychoanalytic theory which emphasizes the denial of castration, does not pay enough attention to the sociological implications. Alfred Adler was better aware of the social differences between the sexes as being a cause of neurotic development. In our society great numbers of men seem to suffer from an inferiority complex "Being half a man," this is one reproach which is more feared than any other. This fear is a powerful motivation towards aggression, and this also applies to the psychiatrist.

Aggressive behavior does have something to do with sex. The rule that the males are the more aggressive of the sexes applies to all mammals. Manly behavior and masculine appearance not only add to sexual attractiveness, but promote chances for social success. Consider, if you will, the fact that every American president elected since 1900 has been the taller of the two competing candidates. Body height is generally considered a distinctive factor, which determines overall male attractiveness.[16] Therefore ample reason exists for men to display their "manly" characteristics. Aggression is one of them and indeed the most outstanding. I propose to name this kind of aggression exhibitionistic aggression. Making a display of one's masculinity, in other words making a show of one's erectness as a male sexual characteristic, is a pathological symptom, whether it be done literally or figuratively.

Aggression, a Phenomenon of Human Encounter

Aggression is never defined by promoting factors alone, it cannot be comprehended when we consider the separate variables of the situation, the victim,

---

[15] M. Fasteau, *The Male Machine* (New York: Dell, 1976).

[16] Glenn Wilson and David Nias, *Love's Mysteries, The Psychology of Sexual Attraction* (London: Open books, 1976).

and the aggressor. We have to consider aggression as a phenomenon of human communication. In the literal sense of the word, aggression means approach. When one person encounters another, there is always something happening; they influence each other. Person A realizes that he is the object which Person B is observing, he himself is a subject for whom B is the object. This is not a purely grammatical question. In every such encounter, we are subject and object, both parties, each in his turn.

When someone feels uneasy about being observed as an object, we might consider him slightly neurotic. However, in so doing, we reduce the existential problem to a psychiatric category. Sartre, in his description of human encounter, did not define psychopathological problems, but human existence.[17] Every encounter is a potential threat. I, a subject, meet another subject, who gives me a place as an object in his world. When I am loved, I am an object, but to me the other person always presents himself as an object, so I regain my subjectivity. I can try to become an object by absolute submission, like a slave. Or I can make the other my object, by caressing him, finally by totally degrading and humiliating. But even this extreme masochism or sadism remains unsatisfying, a failure. In the same way, Merleau-Ponty describes encounter as a relation between master and slave.[18] He, too, did not offer a psychopathological thesis, but depicted human relationships in general terms, and talked about common human problems.

In every communication between people an aggressive factor may be present. They influence one another, and exert power over each other. Surely, this need not lead to violence. Originally, even the word violence did not mean attack. Etymologically, the word violence is akin to the Latin word, *vis*, for force, power. Similarly the German word *Gewalt* is related to the Latin *valeo*: "I am strong." Force and power need not be destructive, and aggression, in the sense of approach, need not be an offensive action. In daily life however, force and power indicate destruction, and every approach implies the threat of attack, of harm being done.

The fate of the words aggression and violence reflects the fate of what man made of the concepts. The theory of aggression as a destructive instinct does not answer the question satisfactorily. No animal ever destroyed other species.[19] The specific position of man is characterized by retarded development, individualization, reflection, self-consciousness, and speech. This grants him abundant possibilities, but also a multitude of risks. These risks include misuse of power, failing communication, and destructive aggression. These are typically human problems.

Biologists can tell us a lot about aggressive behavior in animals, as well as in men. Sexual instincts and the battle for power each play their roles. Ardrey, in his book *The Territorial Imperative*, has stimulated our imaginations on the implications for human behavior. So did Claire and William Russell in *Violence, Monkeys and Men*. Karl Lorenz called his famous book *Das Sogenannte Böse*, "the so-called evil."[20] The English title *On Aggression* does not reflect Lorenz'

[17] Jean-Paul Sartre, *L'être et le Néant* (Paris: Gallimard, 1957).

[18] Maurice Merleau-Ponty, *Phénoménologie de la Perception* (Paris: Gallimard, 1945).

[19] Pierre Teilhard de Chardin, *Le Phénomène Humain* (Paris: Edition du Seuil, 1955).

[20] Karl Lorenz, *On Aggression* (London: Methuen, 1966).

intention, that is, that what we call evil is nothing but a result of man's natural, physiological organization. In biological studies on aggression the sociocultural aspects are often overlooked. It is important to realize that hierarchical struggles in human communities, and territorial difficulties induce human aggression, as they did on Monkey Hill, a rockery crowded with Arabian Baboons at the London Zoo.[21]

In this regard, an outlet for our aggressive drives might be found through adventurous living. Substitutes for hunting attainable to ordinary people are becoming rare in our civilized world, especially in our towns with their constrained areas of greenery imprisoned between slabs of concrete and stone. Criminal behavior seems to be the only opportunity to face danger, to work off one's frustrations, and to act out aggressive instincts. I should not forget to mention, in this context, the possibility of indulging oneself in highway traffic, where aggression and manhunting both seem acceptable and allowable games. Examples of criminal behavior meant to work off our frustrations are not restricted to aggressive crimes, but may be observed in many cases of swindling. The swindler often bears characteristics similar to those of the play sphere. In this play man experiences his freedom; his play also has an aggressive trait. The victim is defeated. Both the swindler and his victim show the tendency to cross the limits, to escape from every day reality into a world of imagination. That is what enables the swindler to deceive others and what makes him a fascinating personality; in literature and mythology the swindler is even worshipped as a hero and a god. He promises enthralling solutions. Even in court and especially when his crimes are published in the newspapers he is sometimes regarded with veneration.

Evil in Man

Evil is not to be explained away by frustration or by any outside circumstances. It seems to be present within man — within every man — as a potential. Ordinary men obediently torture their fellowmen, as Milgram has shown in his experiments.[22] Power tends to corrupt, and absolute power corrupts absolutely, because every man has within him the possibility of the degeneration of all values and of evil. The virtuous citizen is not so very respectable; even the honest psychiatrist does not always deserve the honor and respect which people show him.

Speaking of evil may recall a subject mentioned earlier, the psychiatrist's head of a priest (Heinroth and Guardini). We cannot totally avoid questions of religion and philosophy, when dealing with human disorder. We have to recognize the reality of evil. To some it may seem an easy way of avoiding problems. When psychological and psychiatric attempts for explanation fail, we find recourse in mysticism, and unscientific conceptions. When our reasoning is insufficient, the irrational serves as a makeshift.

We are able to trace a great deal of human misconduct to abnormal brain activities, or to psychological and sociological causes. We make our diagnoses,

[21] Claire and William Russell, *Violence, Monkeys and Man* (London: MacMillan, 1968).
[22] Stanley Milgram, *Obedience to Authority* (New York: Harper & Row, 1974).

organic disorder, psychosis, neurosis, mental deficiency. There are cases however, which do not fit into our psychopathological system. When misbehavior is considered bad we talk of responsibility, imputability, guilt wickedness, evil and sin. One can strike out what does not apply, but each of us uses one or more of these terms. Not only in penal law, but in daily life as well, for we cannot do without these concepts. It would be a very unhuman world, if we could not call each other to account, if we could not blame or praise our fellowman, and if there were no guilt and no merit, if all human conduct were considered the product of causal factors, lying beyond the realm of good and evil. We should not reduce the concept of sin, or a substitute term, to biological, psychological or psychiatric categories. This is one of the main reasons why the psychiatrist should have no intention of acting as a judge. He contributes to the understanding of criminal behavior, but judgment lies beyond his territory.

Acknowledging that some behavior is bad or wicked, we have to accept that aggressive responses are not to be rejected in toto. Criminal behavior requires firm handling. Punishment may be called aggressive, but it ought not to become destructive. Annihilation, e.g., a death-penalty, is no more punishment in the real sense of the word. Punishment is a kind of aggression in the sense of approach; it is an essential mode of contact between people.

If psychiatrists were of the opinion that their categories covered all the bases then they would not and could not cooperate with lawyers, and make their appearance in a penal system in which concepts like guilt, imputability and punishment are taken for granted. They do contribute to this system, however, because they realize that man is more than a product of manifold circumstances, and therefore is essentially answerable, responsible for his doings.

More generally speaking, we might conclude that not every aggression is objectionable, if only we succeed in controlling our destructive tendencies. Likewise, not all human power is objectionable. On the contrary, it should be considered a mandate given us. We should realize our responsibility and our tremendous possibilities. Tremendous seems to be the right word in this context. Our task may cause us to tremble, it may terrify us, but this word "tremendous" also means astonishing, by magnitude, huge. It is a matter of man's vocation.

Man's Vocation

Human behavior is not determined by instincts alone. It results from interaction among a number of variables, including genetic structures, learning patterns, and both physical and social environments. It was formulated in just these words by Annemarie de Waal Malefijt in her interesting anthropological study *Images of Man.*[23] Man is always more than a result of variables. Man is, like the animals, manipulatable, but man is the only creature able to manipulate others.

The role of a poker player, for example, is not suitable when one has to deal with the essential needs and sorrows of one's fellowmen. Man is sometimes too indifferent, or overly careless. He is also often too hostile and aggressive. He

---

[23] Annemarie de Waal Malefijt, *Images of Man* (New York: Knopf, 1974).

may be too premature to judge other people's behavior. These are problems common to both psychiatric practice as well as the execution of penal law. They are also essential problems of humanity as a whole. Central human problems are: human power and its misuse of violence; human encounter and its degeneration to destruction.

We do not exaggerate when we say that in our time these problems have come to a head as never before. Human power has made it possible for us to attain impossibilities. We can now, literally, reach for the moon. But man still behaves rather moonishly, i.e., stupidly. Human communication has made such progress that we can see and hear each other by way of satellites, practically all over our globe. But never has mankind suffered as much from loneliness, never have people lived in such isolation, as they do today. Though we experience so much of each other, we have become more and more estranged, and this estrangement leads to hostility.

Is there a cure for this disease? There are possibilities for the treatment of individual aggression. Psychotherapy has its successes. Some drugs are very useful, and even neurosurgical treatment has introduced new perspectives.[24] The pathology of mankind will not be solved, however, by psychiatry. When Freud was asked by Einstein if there was a way to abolish war, he did not recommend psychoanalytic treatment. He pointed to the power of love, the necessity of promoting more independent thinking, and the development of culture.[25]

Human development and human ingenuity still seems our only hope, but above all love of one's neighbor. Human power remains dangerous; it should be accompanied by justice and love. Power, justice and love are constituents of every human relation, but the three are apt to collide with each other. The increase of human power threatens human existence. The only remedy is to strive towards strengthening the other constituents; justice and love. Great thinkers and philosophers like Guardini, Gabriel Marcel, and Ortega y Gasset have warned against the dehumanization of our world, caused by human development, techniques, and violence. The answer is not psychologic or psychiatric. That would create a society ruled by psychologists, like the *Brave New World* Huxley depicted. The only answer is a call for humanization of man, as Bychowski proposed in his book, *Evil in Man.*[26]

This is what I mean by man's vocation. In following this call, man will have to go his way humbly, submissively. As Gabriel Marcel has put it, the old concept of all religion is that sin means hubris, i.e., overly nurtured pride.[27] He recognizes this pride by the way our techniques control and misuse our planet. He emphasizes the value of being a servant, he praises being plain and unpretentious. In another book Marcel treats the decline of wisdom,[28] and repeatedly emphasizes the need for drawing ourselves together. It is a way of thought al-

---

[24]Vernon H. Mark and Frank R. Erwin, *Violence and the Brain* (New York: Harper & Row, 1970).

[25]Sigmund Freud, "Why War?" (original 1933) in *Civilization, War and Death* (London: The Hogarth Press, 1939).

[26]Gustav Bychowski, *Evil in Man. The Anatomy of Hate and Violence* (New York and London: Grune & Stratton, 1968).

[27]Gabriel Marcel, *Les Hommes centre L'humain* (Paris: La Colombe, 1953).

[28]Gabriel Marcel, *Le déclin de la sagesse* (Paris: Plon, 1957).

ready to be found in Socrates. It is also what the great religions have been concerned with, Buddhism, Judaism, Christianity and Islam; to overcome our self-centeredness.[29] A distinguished psychiatrist, Karl Menninger, reminded us of the reality of sin and the need to conquer our selfishness and pride.[30] Return towards our fellowmen, stepping down from pride to humbleness of mind, from power towards plain service, this will be man's vocation, in this age more needed than ever before. It will also be the only right way in which we can do our jobs as psychiatrists, lawyers, judges or whatever our task may be. There is not much left of the many heads I started with. We are in imminent danger of going out of our heads, of losing control, should we not accept the humble head of a servant. As Christ taught: Whosoever will be great among you, let him be your minister. And whosoever will be chief among you, let him be your servant.[31]

---

[29] Arnold Toynbee: *From Surviving the Future* (Oxford: University Press, 1971).
[30] Karl Menninger: *Whatever Became of Sin?* (New York: Hawthorn Books, 1973).
[31] St. Matthew 20: 26, 27.

Comments on Zeegers' "The Many-Headed Psychiatrist"

Commentator: Ralph Slovenko*

Dr. Michael Zeegers, as I would have expected, has given us a rich and stimulating presentation. Unlike the blind men who described an elephant by the part each touched — one compared it to a snake, another to a tree trunk, and so forth, each giving a truncated observation, Zeegers' presentation is comprehensive. He does not focus on merely one head but on the many heads worn by the psychiatrist — that of physician, king, poker player, priest, judge, police officer, and warrior — and then suggests that "exhibitionistic aggression" underlies the growth of the many heads.

Zeegers, if he had his way, would chop off the head of the psychiatrist who behaves as king, poker player, priest, police officer, or warrior. While Zeegers is speaking metaphorically, it would be appropriate in this symposium on law and psychiatry to observe that as a matter of fact, in every revolution the lawyers are the first to be guillotined. Especially in revolutionary times, lawyers and the law are regarded not as serving society but as exploiting it. "The first thing we have to do," said Shakespeare, "is get rid of the lawyers."

Through the ages, the doctor has not literally "lost his head" because he has been identified as a holy man, sometimes a god. Illness was considered supernaturally caused and supernaturally cured. In Deuteronomy: "I kill and I make alive; I wound and I heal." Invested with the power over life and death, the doctor has been treated with the respect accorded a holy Hindu cow. Throughout history the doctor has been accorded various privileges — with one exception: under the first code of medical ethics, drawn up by the Babylonian king, Hammurabi, "If [the doctor] shall kill the patient or destroy the sight of the eye, his hands shall be cut off." (This was before the A.M.A., so there was no organized protest.) Hippocrates quickly changed things. The doctor gained respect. Under the Hippocratic code, the byword of medical graduates, there is exemption from hard labor: "Physicians," it is said, "should not cut stones." Hippocrates has been called the ideal physician; he believed it was up to nature to do the healing.

The doctor's special status evolved until in late Roman law he and some other professionals were made exempt from all public obligations, including paying taxes and military service.[1] In the middle ages a doctor was not liable for injury to patients unless he inflicted it with evil or criminal intent, whereas other persons were strictly liable for their wrongs.[2] Thereafter, when delictual

---

*Professor of Law and Psychiatry, Wayne State University School of Law, Detroit, Michigan, and author of *Psychiatry and Law* (Boston: Little Brown, 1973).

[1] Justinian's Digest 27.6.2 (vol. 3, p. 123).

[2] A. K. R. Kiralfy and H. Potter (eds.), *Outlines of English Legal History* (London: Sweet & Maxwell, 1958).

responsibility generally became based on intentional or negligent wrongdoing, the halo around the doctor essentially assured him of immunity from suit.

The adulation accorded the doctor continues today, though obviously not with the same intensity. Some years ago, in a social experiment, I happened to wear a doctor's white coat in downtown New Orleans. I found people stepping aside for me as I entered the elevator and that getting a check approved was no hassle. And while just the memory of Elvis Presley's sensuality is a lure to the opposite sex, so too is the doctor's white coat. Marrying a doctor has been the aspiration of many a young girl. One need only recall that every Jewish mother wants her son to be a doctor, and her daughter to marry one. Recently a middle-aged man went into Atlanta's Grady Hospital posing as a heart surgeon; he later said he wanted to attract female companions. The doctor even has a parking place, that most cherished of American prerogatives. During the time I wore the white coat I began to feel as though I were a god — one regarded as a god naturally begins to play the role.

The desire of the psychiatrist to keep the head of the doctor is understandable. Zeegers says we should not behead the psychiatrist's "doctor's head." Medical education, he says, sharpens vision. That may be true; at the same time, the doctor's head is the head that allows the other heads to grow. Realizing this, psychiatrists do not let us forget that they are medical graduates even when they are not acting as doctors. In general, we may note, physicians seem always to use the prefix "Dr." or suffix "M.D." — one might think that it is part of their legal name, but it is not. Consider, for example, the "Report of the Governor's Commission on Individual Privacy to Governor Otis R. Bowen, M.D."[3] The dean of American psychiatry, Dr. Karl A. Menninger, is affectionately known as "Dr. Karl." Thomas Szasz, though he says psychiatry ought not to be cast in the medical model as it deals with problems of living, sometimes has both the prefix "Dr." and the suffix "M.D." surrounding his name.[4] On cross-examination, attorneys are known to throw a doctor off balance by addressing him as "Mister" instead of "Doctor." Just about every psychiatric conference begins with the greeting, "Welcome to this *scientific* meeting," as though they were not sure.

The psychiatrist's "doctor's head," though, is very much in controversy. It may be recalled that in the nineteenth century, medical orientation became almost exclusively somatic. Freud showed the limitation of such a model, and psychiatry resultingly blossomed. It became the clinical discipline within medicine concerned primarily with the study of man and the human condition. In the twentieth century, it became increasingly evident that life circumstances have sweeping implications for illnesses of all kinds. Psychiatry gradually moved very much out of the medical orbit in fact if not in name. But now, threatened by third-party limitations on payment for mental health services, psychiatry is proclaiming a field of activity congruent with the medical model

---

[3] Indianapolis, Indiana, Dec. 1, 1976.

[4] One psychiatrist suggests that it would be a good idea to distinguish in print, as done in Europe, between doctors of medicine (psychiatrists) and other "doctors" by referring to M.D.s as "Dr. med. so and so." Ltr., *Psychiatric News*, Jan. 20, 1978, p. 13.

of disease. Some spokesmen for psychiatry say that it has strayed into unfamiliar terrain by focusing on social and community mental health problems, and declare that its medical identity is in jeopardy. Editorials in psychiatric journals emphasize the necessity for psychiatrists to "remedicalize." Such a path would, however, be a retreat to a limited model of diseases.[5]

The subject matter of psychiatry is not disease in any commonly understood meaning of the term, but rather involves problems of biopsychosocial adjustment. Wearing the mantel of the doctor, it is very easy for the psychiatrist to go riding off in all directions. But where is the boundary of the psychiatrist *qua* doctor? One psychiatrist puts it: "Psychiatrists are having a devil of a time cutting out a territory they can call their own between psychologists who can do psychotherapy better and internists who know more about drugs. And nowadays there are so many other holy men and gurus that the psychiatrist as holy man seems weak by comparison."[6]

The first part of Zeegers' paper hangs together on the hydra analogy; the second part on man's aggression. The link between the two parts is what Zeegers calls "exhibitionistic aggression." The "ego trip," as it may also be called, begins noticeably in medical school. It is, he says, and rightly we think, that which prompts the doctor or psychiatrist to grow so many heads. In considerable measure, other "experts" (to the extent allowed them) do the same. Then again, who does not become aggressive given the opportunity? Socrates said that the artisan, though he may know his trade, does not know the boundaries of his knowledge. The learned Greek further observed: "Experts suffer from swelled heads. They offer testimony outside their realm." "Expansiveness is not inherently undesirable," though, says one psychiatrist (speaking about women today). "I see it as part of the self-actualizing process of healthy growth and autonomy."[7] As Zeegers says, not every aggression is disagreeable.

Zeegers in his essay associates himself with Lord Acton's admonition — power corrupts, and absolute power corrupts absolutely — and Alfred Adler's psychology of man constructed on the theme of power. We might say in response; weakness corrupts, and absolute weakness corrupts absolutely. In the words of Erich Fromm, "The lust of power is not rooted in strength."[8] It is rooted in weakness. Everyone has an Achilles' heel, real or imagined; and everyone attempts to compensate for it in some way or other. Adler in his work pointed out the effects of "organ inferiorities" — that is, congenitally weak or poorly functioning organs — on personality development. Just as the body reacts to repair its weaknesses, Adler suggested that this process of compensation also

[5] George L. Engel, "The Need for a New Medical Model: A Challenge for Biomedicine," *Science* 196 (1977):129.

[6] Communication of December 20, 1977, from Dr. R. E. Reinert, Hospital Director, Veterans Administration Hospital, St. Cloud, MN.

[7] Dr. Alexandra Symonds, quoted in "Women and Success — Why Some Find It So Painful," *New York Times,* Jan. 28, 1978, p. 14.

[8] Quoted in Arnold A. Hutschnecker, "The Lessons of Eagleton," *New York Times,* Oct. 30, 1972, p. 31. "Power can mean power *over* people, or it can mean power to do things. What the sadist is striving for is power *over* people, precisely because he lacks the power *to be*." Erich Fromm, *The Anatomy of Human Destructiveness* (New York: Holt, Rinehart & Winston, 1973), p. 330.

proceeds in the psychological sphere.[9] The term "homeostasis" can be used to refer to mental functioning as well as physiological processes. Menninger calls homeostasis the achieving of "vital balance" — in ordinary language, staying on one's rocker.[10]

Often by psychological means, Adler claimed an overcompensation may be brought about. Beethoven, suffering from congenital ear disease, composed beautiful music. Milton, in his blindness, wrote magnificent literature. Demosthenes, a childhood stutterer, became one of the greatest orators. On the other hand, where nature fails to produce a correction, pathological processes — inability, neurosis, isolation — may be set in motion to put things in balance.

The same "vital balance" principle within the individual that has the capacity for maintaining physiological functioning under constantly changing conditions of life is also applied to the balanced functioning of the mind and the dynamic equilibrium of the individual with his social environment. The adjustive techniques used by the mind are so systematized that they are indeed called mental defense mechanisms. They are lucidly discussed by Anna Freud in her book, "The Ego and Mechanisms of Defense."[11] Some of these mechanisms of defense, ways of reacting, are compensation, rationalization, idealization, reaction formation, and displacement.

In infancy one is impressed by bigness, and thereafter the impression has its psychological effects. To children, grownups are like giants; and one of the first and hardest tasks in childhood is to get up on one's feet. This childhood experience of inferiority and helplessness generates a drive to prove one's significance, or "bigness," in any way one can. Christian scholars established that Adam was nearly 124 feet in height. He must have been the size of Jack's Giant. For children the primary source of confusion is scale, as Jonathan Swift and Lewis Carroll both make quite clear. The impression made by bigness promotes the big person's chances for success. Height inspires veneration. Zeegers goes so far as to claim that every American President elected since 1900 has been the taller of the two competing candidates. The elected candidate may not actually have been the taller but it probably seemed that way. In actual fact, Gerald Ford is taller than Jimmy Carter but "headbumping clumsiness" plagued Ford; Carter's managers were very much concerned by his relative shortness. Franklin Roosevelt, an invalid, made efforts to stand but he compensated by his reassuring voice at fireside chats.

No dwarf was ever elected President of the United States, on that we can all agree. There may be prejudices against blacks and women and others, but there is also prejudice against short people and dwarves. The small boy is called "Peewee," "Small Change," "Shrimp." A national organization of 2,000 members,

---

[9] Alfred Adler, *Study of Organ Inferiority and Its Psychical Compensation: Contribution to Clinical Medicine,* tr. Smith E. Jeliffe (Nervous & Mental Disease Monographs: No. 24), 1917. See also Maggie Scarf, *Body, Mind, Behavior* (Washington, D.C.: New Republic, 1976), p. 123; William S. Walsh, *The Inferiority Feeling* (New York: Dutton, 1928).

[10] Karl Menninger, *The Vital Balance/The Life Process in Mental Health and Illness* (New York: Viking, 1963).

[11] Anna Freud, *The Ego and the Mechanism of Defense* (New York: International Universities Press, 1967). See also George E. Vaillant, "Understanding and Profiting from Ego Defense Mechanisms," *New York Times,* Feb. 25, 1978, p. 21.

"The Little People of America," along with scores of irate callers in several cities recently successfully persuaded radio stations to stop playing singer-writer Randy Newman's song "Short People." Among other slurs the song says, "Short people got no reason to live." The song uses words like "grubby" and "stubby" and "peep-peep-peep" to describe short people.

"Shape-*up*" if you want a job. One executive of a major corporation says: "The most frequent question I'm asked is 'How do I get promoted?' My answer: 'The easiest way is to be born right and be born tall.' (Corporate officers are at least two inches taller than the average male.) Now that doesn't mean shorter men and those of less august lineage can't make it to the top of the batting order. It just means that they have to be better at what they do . . . or communicate better or think smarter."[12]

And one way up is "exhibitionistic aggression," as Zeegers calls it. Everyone feels shortsighted, and they try to compensate (and sometimes overcompensate). For a certain kind of man, the thought that anyone can literally "look down on him" is insufferable. Stalin at Teheran was furious when he was seated lower than Roosevelt and Churchill; he got his chair raised. In Charlie Chaplin's "The Great Dictator," there is a barber-chair scene in which Hitler and Mussolini each tries to pump himself higher than the other. Harry Cohn, when he dined out, placed a telephone book on his chair.

Just after reading Zeegers' paper, as I was checking out of a hotel from a conference, a Harvard law professor (over 6-foot-5), towering over others almost like a giraffe, chiseled a little ahead of the line. A young woman blurted out, "Have you noticed! Tall people tend to be arrogant, and small people compliant." But as she said this, she pushed ahead of the line. She confronted him; and she used his tactic. The lanky professor actually said he felt "belittled." Also at this conference just about every woman there, in a turnabout, was smoking a pipe or cigar (a cigar is not just a smoke, said Freud); not a male was (they were wearing narrow ties or none at all).[13] Today, fewer tall women are wearing flats or slumping their shoulders. Women's liberation too manifests itself by the image of bigness and power. Women now want to get "ahead" faster.

A person who feels himself helpless to control his fate may unconsciously choose crime rather than mental collapse because breaking the law can give a liberating sense of power. "During the planning and execution of a criminal act," says Halleck, "the offender is a free man. He is immune from the oppressive dictates of others since he has temporarily broken out of their control."[14] Yochelson and Samenow in their study of the "criminal personality" say:

> The pursuit of power and control pervades the criminal's thinking, conversation, and action. Power and control are sought in irrespon-

---

[12] Gerard R. Roche, "Restarting a Stalled Executive," *American Way* (inflight magazine of American Airlines), Jan. 1978, p. 49.

[13] Jane Trahey's recent book on "Women and Power" is advertised, "If you crave that great reward – power – then grab this book, read it, and learn its lessons well." Jane Trahey, *Women and Power* (New York: Rawson, 1978).

[14] Quoted in *New York Times*, Dec. 18, 1977, p. E-8. The thesis is developed in Seymour L. Halleck, *Psychiatry and the Dilemmas of Crime: A Study of Causes, Punishment and Treatment* (Berkeley: University of California Press, 1971).

sible ways purely for self-aggrandizement. The criminal approaches life, pursuing personal triumphs, conquests and build-ups. To achieve these, he promotes himself at the expense of others. He recognizes no limit to his personal power and control; the world is his to do with as he pleases. Whatever he does, whomever he deals with, he expects the world to adapt immediately to his wants, even when he is apprehended and confined.[15]

The swindler is indeed worshipped in the manner that he breaks rules.

"Every man would like to be God, if it were possible," said Bertrand Russell. Getting up in the world, literally or figuratively speaking, indicates a position of more dignity than "down." Highborn is up, lowborn is down. High is heaven, low is hell. One gets a "dressing down." "Grow up" is a tall order. "Catch up." "Bottoms up," proves you're a man. The cobra, although a venomous snake, is worshipped by some people as divine, and that is because it has the ability to rise at will (like a young man's penis). "Put *up,* or shut up," we say. Some men still believe that height has something to do with the size of the penis, despite assurances to the contrary from Masters and Johnson.

Pride is the emotional stature of a person, and it expresses itself bodily. The more upright a person, the more we admire him. A speaker who slouches on a lectern is not as compelling as one who stands erect and unsupported. Praise is for the up-standing and out-standing. The symbol of victory in a match is being held aloft, and the victor's hand goes upward. Subjectively, upness means being up in self-esteem. We say that someone has developed a "swelled head" or "big head" because of his success; the individual in question actually perceives his head as larger. The man in public office ("his Worship") begins to walk about so upright that one might think he were a God. The public's adulations and ovations take the place of mother love, and fill his body, sometimes it seems, almost to the bursting point.[16] Body language experts say that love makes you appear taller, walk more erect. Man expresses defeat, on the other hand, by a head bent downward; he feels deflated. The beaten dog hangs its tail between its legs.

To increase the effect of physical stature, chieftains wore towering headgear, and kings seated themselves on an elevated throne and wore a crown. He was called, "Your *High*ness," and people bowed before him kissing his foot. The Jews speak of High Holy Days and standard English has the expression "high days and holidays." Melvin Belli, the flamboyant trial lawyer, wears high heels (and named his son "Caesar"). In a courtroom, the judge sits on an elevated bench. The implicit message: "You are higher than I am, therefore you are dominant." We have such expressions as "kiss the dirt," "bite the dust."

---

[15] Samuel Yochelson and Stanton E. Samenow, *The Criminal Personality* (New York: Jason Aronson, 1977), vol. 2, p. 6. Houston housewife desperado Sylvia Jean Brown got tired of tending house and raising children. Looking for something more to her life, she chose a .38 caliber pistol, a .45-caliber automatic, and a sawed-off shotgun. She got away with a series of holdups, she said, because "my femininity is the element of surprise." It gave her "a complete, natural high, a feeling of knowing I could do it. It was power." "It's too bad there is no legal way people can live like this" she said. AP and UPI news-release, *Detroit Free Press,* Feb. 11, 1978, p. 7-C.

[16] Arnold A. Hutschnecker, *The Drive for Power* (New York: Evans, 1974).

Christ's ascension has never ceased to fascinate man. In the rock opera production, "Jesus Christ Superstar," Christ is asked, "Do you think you could get much higher?" In the psychoanalytic situation the analysand is put down on the couch (and he regresses to childhood experiences); his task is to get up. Employment services or agencies commonly have the name "Apex" or "Zenith." A man keeps *up* with the Jones's, and he wants a *raise*. The struggle to "stay on top" is another phrase that refers to potency as well as the sexualization of the business world. The *Wall Street Journal* advertises that it is written "to help you go higher."

King Kong is not called King for nothing; he did not idly choose the Empire State Building, this highest of high-rise buildings. In a meditation on King Kong, Bernard writes: "We want King to grow big and approach the blond maiden with bloodshot, lustful eyes. . . . Exactly how big *is* Kong's penis? It is a matter of monumental cultural and psychological interest. And a great mystery: for Kong' penis is never shown. . . . [Is it] the size of the Empire State Building?"[17] But Kong could not live erect in the New World, and uttering a last terrifying cry from his battered heart, he falls.

Are we hearing an anguished cry from psychiatrists as well as from other physicians? We used to think that one way to be a God is to be a doctor, but increasingly people no longer feel awed or intimidated by the doctor. More and more, individuals are seeking to subtract the value of their time spent waiting to see the doctor from his bill.[18] Now, not only psychiatry in particular but also medicine in general is challenged in, and scorned for, its claims of expertness. Medicine itself is on the critical list; down it is going. We hear it said: "The surgeon is one who knows nothing and does everything, the psychiatrist is one who knows everything and does nothing."

The doctor's head as priest, we may say, has been replaced by the head of a businessman, a head unmentioned by Zeegers. When one visits the doctor today, one feels that he is in a business establishment. The medical clinic has the air of Wall Street. With the businessman's head, will the doctor be able to grow as many heads as was possible when he was identified as a priest? Not likely.[19] Increasingly, the autonomy of the doctor is being curtailed by malpractice suits, licensing and certification laws, and general monitoring of his work. Increasingly, the medical profession is being compared to the mafia. The medical profession does not follow the rules of the marketplace yet makes a bundle out of it. The fees and costs in insurance programs are leading to demands that the doctor be put on a fixed salary. (It was Plato's fantasy to have a total subjugation of the profession's autonomy.) Leon Eisenberg, Harvard psychiatrist, recently observed, "Whereas doctors were once thought to be more humane than

[17] Kenneth Bernard, "King Kong: A Meditation," *New American Review* 14 (1972): 182, at 185. "King Kong" was Hitler's favorite movie. John Leonard, "Mr. Fiedler's Sideshow," *New York Times*, Feb. 21, 1978, p. 33.

[18] Ralph Charell, *How to Get the Upper Hand* (New York: Stein & Day, 1978), p. 19.

[19] Max Lerner puts it thus: "Most of all, the cause for the loss of credibility of the medical profession lies in its commercialization — the 'bottom line' morality taken over from business enterprise." Forward to Edgar Berman, *The Solid Gold Stethoscope* (New York: Macmillan, 1976), p. x.

lawyers and judges, the obverse seems to hold today.[20] Actually, in a general way, all of the professions are under fire. The public is becoming especially suspicious of the elite and the professionals.[21]

The Bible teaches, "The greater thou art, the more humble thou art." Unless one is God, it seems that it is through humility that one saves his head. This is Zeegers' message.

[20] Quoted in *Psychiatric News*, Jan 6, 1978, p. 37. Movies like "The Hospital" (countless slipups result in the deaths of doctors and nurses as well as patients), "Such Good Friends" (a patient who dies from simple cosmetic surgery), and "Coma" (malevolent forces in a Boston hospital cause a number of patients to go into coma) contrast sharply with "Marcus Welby" (a kindly country-type doctor who even made house calls). Joe Baltake, "Dr. Kildare Would Probably Faint," *Detroit Free Press*, Feb. 18, 1978, p. 11.

[21] "Never trust a lawyer, banker or politician, in or out of office – in fact, take action in reverse to such advice." Ray L. Trautman, educator, quoted in Israel Shenker, "Who's Who in America Talk About What's What in Life," *New York Times*, Feb. 15, 1978, p. 39.

Comments on Zeeger's "The Many-Headed Psychiatrist"

Commentator: David N. Weisstub*

Dr. Zeegers, in his address on "The Many-Headed Psychiatrist," has brought to the attention of a wide audience of psychiatrists, lawyers and theologians a humanistic analysis of the role of the psychiatrist, particularly in the field of forensic science. In his remarks, Professor Zeegers has entered the debate about the proper definition of the psychiatrists' relationship to values such as liberty, and about its complex relations with the criminal sanction process. He contends that we should not expect the psychiatrist to be pre-defined or given a uni-dimensional function that will pre-empt his professional life from bearing the burdens placed upon him by the accidents of history.

According to Zeegers we should not retreat in the face of antipsychiatric literature to bombard the psychiatric community with the criticism that the physician is the inapplicable type around which to model psychiatry; or in the alternative to suggest the psychiatrist, even if we do admit his proper place as the physician, cannot achieve the level of scientific certitude associated with the medical model. Although there are difficulties in developing a classification system as tight as the codification of crime (which we know incidentally to be rife with fuzziness), we must be cautious, he implies, not to throw the baby out with the bath water. The language of symptoms represents a signpost for human responses based on knowledge of a professional nature. In and of itself, our belief that the psychiatrist is predominantly a doctor with the responsibility of offering a professional service, should not be a premise to be abandoned in searching for a theory of function and role. Rather, he asserts that we should begin from that standpoint and then explore the extent to which other functions may be in conflict with that archetypal characteristic.

The person perceived as a healer will likely be treated by some as infallible and monarchical in his prescriptions. In contemporary discussions about the crisis of science in psychiatry, which concentrates in part on its inability to establish proper scientific criteria for its social decisions, the psychiatrist may rightly be described as a de-throned monarch. In response to this crisis of status, the psychiatrist, as Professor Zeegers rightly points out, may have a tendency to play a hard game of poker, disguising the degree to which he is inadequate in terms of what society expects of him. It is imperative that when psychiatry plays roulette or deals a "heavy hand" that it be arrested unless, of

*Professor of Law, Osgoode Hall Law School of York University, Downsview, Ontario, Canada; and Editor-in-Chief, *International Journal of Law and Psychiatry*.

course, we have accepted the morality of gambling and the odds are not stacked. This is rare in instances where the psychiatrist and the client are in unequal bargaining positions.

Professor Zeegers indicates that the mythological or religious dimensions of psychiatry have been well-worn in history and that psychiatry deals with a range of human problems about which a great deal of intellectual history has been organized. It is in this area of discovering the basis upon which psychiatry functions as a social ordering process that psychiatry may now have a great deal to offer. The area of forensic psychiatry is especially compelling as a testing ground for the parameters of psychiatric practice because in its work it cannot escape from sharing responsibility with the priest and the judge. Deviant behavior is deeply connected to the contexts of social description which reflect specific cultures, and at various periods in history what is allowable into the domain of psychiatry is the result of a subtle give and take which occurs among the respective professions. We assume that the priest operates against the background of a set of cosmological or myth-oriented symbols which in a mysterious way dictate the nature of religious life. It is natural then that psychiatrists will be guarded in making claims about psychiatric priesthoods except in the limited sense of acknowledging that psychiatry is believed in as a system of individual and social prescriptions.

Zeegers takes the position that the psychiatrist "should not play the role of a priest" and should avoid any attempt at magic-making. There is a necessity however, in his view, for psychiatry to confront the spiritual ramifications of the human condition in order to avoid falling into the trap of treating the human being in isolation from his life crises. Here Professor Zeegers has indeed raised a dilemma. For if psychiatry is to embrace its own mythologies and yet also expand its orientation to see the relationship between its various theories or beliefs about the nature of man, while still stressing the limitations of science and a rigid positivistic medical model, will it not find it extremely difficult to delineate the precise boundaries of its theory, authority, and function from those of theology? The psychiatric hydra is a puzzling phenemon, containing paradoxes and impasses which are irresolvable. Could it be the nature of the beast that not only are the heads difficult to separate one from the other but also that the eradication of any of its parts may produce a swallowing up of the function of the destroyed member in a fashion which is not immediately apparent?

This problem is accentuated in psychiatry's relationship with the judging function. If the judicial system takes pains to accept absolute jurisdiction over decision making there is the tendency to rely very heavily on psychiatric input to the point where commentators have asserted that psychiatry has usurped legal responsibility and *de facto* taken over both the determination of insanity in civil and criminal matters, and the exercise of judicial discretion in areas such as sentencing and probation. If we choose another route and place lawyers on panels with psychiatrists and laypersons to advise or decide on insanity, the difficulty is created of not knowing which criteria are critical and binding. The distinctions that Dr. Zeegers has drawn between judge and psychiatrist are most certainly in accord with our conventional wisdom in law. Nonetheless, we should recognize that while in theory the law has supremacy, the fact that we are indeed dealing with an unwieldy hydra has meant that, in practice, it is difficult to know who is exercising supremacy at any given time.

In discussing the policing and soldiering aspects of psychiatry Dr. Zeegers has alerted us to the importance of sorting out external and internal forces which press upon psychiatry, often resulting in a wedge being driven between the patient and a human delivery of psychiatric care or assessment. Psychiatrists are placed in a position of effective control over their clients and often for complex reasons display aggressive and ambivalent behavior towards them. Dr. Zeegers suggests that psychiatrists might, on occasion, compensate for their attributed sensitivity by exerting needless force in their conduct. This is an intriguing perception and one which I believe could be applied as well to the professional community of lawyers. Lawyers are expected to behave aggressively and it has been observed by some that the preponderance of lawyers in political and corporate affairs underscores the correlation of law and power. It is broadly accepted in industrial societies that the personality types of psychiatrists and lawyers are likely opposites. This contributes to anxieties about professional and social performance which undoubtedly frustrate the sensible goal of breaking down professional stereotypes.

Professor Zeegers has dealt directly with the problem of evil. He argues that man's evil cannot be reduced to biological or psychiatric categories. In his view, man must explore his aggressive faculties in order to get in touch with his instinct for revenge and for manipulation of others, since his rationality gives him a special potentiality for structured evil. Psychiatry has the power to order and punish the vulnerable and the outcast. Because it also carries the magic of knowing the unconscious, it may impose itself on the law with the air of both objectivity and humanism. Zeegers has told us in a provocative and yet thoughtful manner that in learning about its many roles we might be in an improved position to prevent the manufacture of evil.

On the other side there is a legal hydra which, since the birth of psychiatry, has been leading a clandestine existence with the creature that Zeegers has described. At this point in history there are undoubtedly offspring of these relationships which make the job of regulating hydras a confusing social task. It will not help us to believe that they do not exist. Although it may offend our aesthetic sense we should be prepared to welcome these hydras and in keeping company with them learn to accept them while subduing their threatening attributes.

The Limits of Psychiatric Authority

Jonas Robitscher*

Psychiatrists have great authority — more than they realize — and their authority is constantly growing greater. Until recently little attention has been paid to the expansion of psychiatric authority, and now when there is a developing psychiatric literature on the subject much of it is devoted to (a) criticisms of psychiatrists concerning the abuse of psychiatric power in countries such as Russia on the ground that it is used to enforce ideology; or (b) abuse of psychiatric power in the quasi-criminal field in which treatment holdings are imposed on those accused of criminal acts who meet novel diagnostic criteria of such conditions as sexual psychopathy or defective delinquency. Psychiatrists have become aware that there has been a wider attack on psychiatric authority by non-psychiatrists, particularly sociologists and lawyers, and a few "anti-psychiatric" psychiatrists. But most psychiatrists tend to think of abuses as infrequent, occurring for the most part in other countries, and at home confined to special situations — with which they are not involved and they discount the criticisms because of their sources. Most psychiatrists have not attempted to conceptualize the great extension of authority which has accrued to them and they do not concern themselves with its appropriate limits. Some setting of limits has been undertaken by courts, particularly in the field of commitment and the rights of hospitalized patients, but for the most part psychiatric authority has continued to be ill-defined, without effective limitation, not recognized by psychiatrists for its abusive potential, and not sufficiently monitored by the legal system.

Definitions

The question of the "uses and abuses" of psychiatry is now beginning to come to the fore, partly because of the burgeoning of a legal and sociological literature which equates psychiatry with other agents of social control. So we are forced at this time to start to come to terms with the topic of the limits of psychiatric authority. When we work with the subject we find that the limits are extraordinarily difficult to set. Other branches of medicine, other social institutions are easier to deal with; the authority of another kind of doctor, the authority of a judge is easier to define, but psychiatry (among its other strange attributes) mixes features of both medical and legal authority and as a result enjoys powers that go with both disciplines that are not usually combined.

Before we can define the limits of psychiatric authority, we must define psy-

*Henry R. Luce Professor of Law and the Behavioral Sciences, Emory University, Atlanta, Georgia. This paper continues and amplifies arguments made in Dr. Robitscher's Isaac Ray Award Lecture Series, "The Uses and Abuses of Psychiatry," given at George Washington University, Washington, D.C., October, 6–8, 1977; the lectures and panel discussion that made up that series appear in *Journal of Psychiatry and Law* 5 nos. 3 and 4 (1977).

chiatry and psychiatrist. The glossary of the American Psychiatric Association gives us a definition of psychiatry that does not begin to encompass all the activities that go on in the name of psychiatry: it says psychiatry is "the medical science that deals with the origin, diagnosis, prevention, and treatment of mental disorders."[1] The definition is inadequate because much that goes into modern psychiatry is not medical and is not scientific and because psychiatry deals with many mental states and conditions which are not truly mental disorders. The term "mental disorder" is defined officially as a psychiatric illness or disease included in the approved classification schemes of the World Health Organization and the American Psychiatric Association,[2] but the fact that many conditions not previously listed have been included in the draft of the next edition of the APA Diagnostic and Statistical Manual and other conditions have been or are proposed for delisting indicates that the field of psychiatry cannot be simply defined by saying it deals only with mental disorders as delineated by the World Health Organization or the American Psychiatric Association.

The preliminary report of President Carter's Commission on Mental Health defined "America's mental health problem" as "not limited to those individuals with disabling mental illness and identified psychiatric disorders. It also includes those people who suffer the effects of . . . societal ills which . . . affect their everyday lives."[3] Since there is no one who does not feel the effects of societal ills which affect everyday life, the definition includes the totality of the people as the psychiatric population. A recent article on community psychiatry, not untypically, gives a similarly broad and vague definition of the population to be treated. The author suggests that because of the difficulty in defining "mental disorder," we can use the pragmatic definition of "those problems which are presently referred to mental health personnel." He continues: "These problems may or may not fit discrete diagnostic categories, but will, generally involve difficulties in thought perceptions, feelings, and/or behavior."[4] Once psychiatric problems were defined narrowly; now they are defined very broadly. Most of us although conscious that psychiatrists — at least in their role as value-setters and definers of normality — affect every phase of society would still not define the mental health problem or the scope of legitimate psychiatric authority as broadly as the President's Commission or the author of the article did, but we all must concede that psychiatry has become more than the medical specialty dealing with seriously abnormal mental states.

Some evidence for the fact that psychiatry has overrun its borders is our inability to confine the term "psychiatric" and "psychiatrist." People in psychiatric care are receiving treatment which may be given by psychologists, social workers, or members of other disciplines — or by someone not a member of any discipline at all — and when they are in a psychiatric hospital, a great majority of the therapists and staff with whom they have contact will be performing psychiatric functions but will not be psychiatrists.

---

[1] American Psychiatric Association, *A Psychiatric Glossary,* 4th ed. (Washington, D.C.: APA, 1975).
[2] *Id.*
[3] "Preliminary Report of the President's Commission on Mental Health," Sept. 1, 1977, Washington, D.C., p. 2.
[4] Ricardo F. Muñoz, "The Primary Prevention of Psychiatric Problems," *Community Mental Health Review* 1, no. 6 (1976): 1, 5–15.

When I speak of psychiatry and psychiatrists, I am using these terms in this modern expanded sense; I am not only talking about the authority exercised by physicians who have taken a three year accredited residency in psychiatry but the authority of all those who make psychiatric decisions.

At one time psychiatry was easy to define; it was indeed that medical discipline dealing with abnormal mental states. A second root of modern psychiatry developed in the early century — Freudian psychoanalytic psychiatry which represented a more psychological, although not an academic psychological, approach. In 1958 when Hollingshead and Redlich wrote *Social Class and Mental Illness,* they could say there were two kinds of practitioners, the Directive and Organic practitioners who were the inheritors of the more strictly medical tradition and the Analytic and Psychological practitioners who had brought into psychiatry Freudian and other nonmedical material and attitudes.[5]

Since then we have seen the development of behavior modification, springing from the more traditional psychology, which brings into psychiatry entirely new concepts and new techniques of treatment. We have also seen a variety of new therapies practiced by a variety of new mental health professions. The list of therapeutic approaches now includes psychoanalysis, psychoanalytic psychotherapy, existential analysis, direct analysis, milieu therapy, Rogerian therapy, humanistic psychology as developed by Maslow, Gestalt therapy, Reichian bioenergetics, primal therapy, the mysticotranscendental approaches, group therapies including psychodrama and transactional analysis, family therapy, network therapy, crisis intervention therapy, behavioral-directive approaches including chemotherapy and other somatic therapies and the behavior therapies, and biofeedback. I am listing only primary therapies; there are a number of additional therapies — art therapy, occupational therapy, recreational therapy, dance therapy, vocational therapy and more — which deserve inclusion as ancillary therapies.

We have opened the boundaries of our discipline so wide that that when we use the terms "psychiatrist" and "psychiatric treatment" we include practitioners who are not formal psychiatrists, clinical psychologists, or psychoanalysts; we include social workers, registered nurses, practical nurses, counselors, pastoral counselors, ex-addicts and ex-alcoholics and other indigenous workers, and a large category we term "mental health technicians" to indicate a lack of advanced professional training. All these people enjoy psychiatric authority; they all make "psychiatric decisions."[6]

Should we define psychiatrist as anyone who works on the problems of mental disease? But we have said there is no accepted or acceptable definition of mental disease. A committee of the American Psychiatric Association for the past several years has been working on definitions of "psychiatry" and "mental illness"; the length of time they have taken in their deliberations suggests

---

[5] August Hollingshead and Frederick Redlich, *Social Class and Mental Illness* (New York: Wiley, 1958), 155–161.

[6] For a description of the varied backgrounds of mental health personnel at one community mental health center, see E. Mansell Pattison, Donald A. Hackenberg, Ellis Wayne, and Paul Wood, "A Code of Ethics for a Community Mental Health Program," *Hospital and Community Psychiatry* 27 (1976): 29–32, 30.

the difficulties they are having. And when it announces the final definitions, there is little chance that they will be accepted without argument.

I have not tried to define psychiatry or psychiatrist but I have made it clear that we are speaking about a field which is large, amorphous, and is surely more than merely a specialized branch of medicine. I have indicated the breadth of the field and the diversity of the people who make psychiatric decisions.

What Kinds of Decisions do These "Psychiatrists" Make?

I think it is helpful to devise a rough classification of psychiatric decision-making and the kind of compulsion that it exerts on patients and others. First, there is the distinction between implicit and explicit authority. Much of what a psychiatrist does with his patient — and much of what psychiatric authority does for society by its definitions of normality and abnormality — has no enforcing mechanism; its authority stems from the willingness of the patient or some other social grouping to conform to psychiatric expectations, to abide by psychiatric rules; this implicit authority is dependent on the prestige of psychiatry which leads to the acceptance of psychiatric pronouncements. Explicit psychiatric authority has enforcing mechanisms; the psychiatrist who determines that a sexual psychopath is not safe to be released to society is exerting authority that cannot be evaded or even easily contested.

Then there are various categories of psychiatric decision-making in terms of whether the authority is specific — exerted on the individual — or general — exerted on groups by defining their norms and expectations.

Implicit psychiatric authority is the hardest to conceptualize, but it is nevertheless very real. An anxious patient submits to psychiatric authority because he sees the psychiatrist as an expert and a source of help; the pychiatrist then has the power to intervene into the "personal life-space" of that individual. The psychiatrist is sometimes subtly directive; sometimes he is not subtle; he may use threats of the termination of treatment if the patient does not conform; he imposes his values systems, often well considered and meant to be helpful but not necessarily the patient's own. Freud's patient known as the Wolfman, because a temporary neurosis of early childhood had centered about a fear of wolves, in recent years has written about Freud's direction to him in the early years of his analysis, around 1910:

> I would have married Therese then and there, had this not been contrary to the rule Professor Freud had made that a patient should not make any decision which would irreversibly influence his later life. If I wanted to complete my treatment with Freud successfully, it was necessary for me to follow his rule whether I wanted to or not.[7]

In 1924 in her novel, *Mrs. Dalloway,* Virginia Woolf desribes a fictional Harley Street psychiatrist — based on her own encounters with psychiatrists who had treated her for suicidal psychotic depressions. Sir William Bradshaw was controlling and directive; he advised "proportion, divine proportion in all

---

[7]The Wolf-man, "Memoirs of the Wolf-man, 1909–1911," *Bull. of the Phila. Association for Psycho-analysis* 19 (1969): 183–196, 195.

things,"[8] just as a real life Harley Street specialist had advised, "Equanimity — equanimity — practice equanimity, Mrs. Woolf."[9] Sir William Bradshaw went so far as to advise his patients whether or not they should have children, just as real life practitioners had advised Virginia Woolf. She wrote of Sir William:

> You invoke proportion; order rest in bed; rest in solitude; silence and rest, rest without friends, without books, without messages; six months' rest; until a man who went in weighing seven stone six comes out weighing twelve. . . .
>
> Worshipping proportion, Sir William not only prospered himself but made England prosper, secluded her lunatics, forbade childbirth, penalised despair, made it impossible for the unfit to propagate their views until they, too, shared his sense of proportion.[10]

Recently Janet Gotkin, who has vividly described her ten-year history as a patient in *Too Much Anger, Too Many Tears*, has written that in spite of the serious symptoms she suffered — delusions, hallucination, terrors, suicidal gestures, a serious suicide attempt — she feels that she was done an injustice, and prevented from making the progress of which she was capable, by her therapist's refusal to allow her to experience depression and to see her feelings of alienation as legitimate. "Little by little," she wrote, "I ripped away the facade of jargon and mystification and saw that out of my pain and groping the doctors had produced a mental patient, unable to survive anywhere but in a so-called mental hospital."[11]

Many patients feel extreme gratitude for the interventions of their doctors, which for the most part are well-intentioned, at least on a conscious level. (On a less conscious level the psychiatrist may feel a need to control or countertransference hostility.) But even grateful willing patients are being subjected to psychiatric authority. When the patient is a well-functioning neurotic seeing the psychiatrist of his own free will and well enough integrated to be free to leave the relationship if the psychiatrist becomes too authoritarian in ways that seem imperiling, then the coercive aspect of psychotherapy never needs to surface. With more anxious and more uncontrolled patients, dependency and the threat of possible commitment become the lever for the exerting of psychiatric authority. There are other levers too. During my psychiatric residency I knew one voluntary patient who was told by her admitting doctor that if she persisted in insisting on leaving the hospital he would be forced to recommend to her family that she receive a lobotomy! Patients are sometimes given electroconvulsive therapy to prevent their signing out against advice.

The Power of Commitment

Probably the main source of psychiatric authority is the power to commit people and to detain them in psychiatric hospitals — so-called "civil" or "civilian"

---

[8] Virginia Woolf, *Mrs. Dalloway* (New York: Harcourt, 1949), p. 149.

[9] Leonard Woolf, *Downhill All the Way* (New York: Harcourt, Brace and World, 1967), p. 51.

[10] Virginia Woolf, *supra*, note 8.

[11] Janet Gotkin and Paul Gotkin, *Too Much Anger, Too Many Tears* (New York: Quadrangle, 1975), p. 382.

mental hospitals and also hospitals for the criminally insane. The power to commit was formerly strictly a judicial power, but legislatures have delegated the power to commit to psychiatrists through the instrumentalities of medical and administrative commitment, and although these procedures allow recourse to the courts, the patient is effectively under the control of psychiatric authority unless he can prove that the commitment is patently not warranted. In recent years we have seen a swing in some United States jurisdictions back from the liberal administrative and medical commitment system to a more judicially protected system,[12] but even in these jurisdictions there continues to be almost complete reliance on the psychiatric expertise to support the commitment; most of the power remains with the psychiatrist. Although the physician-psychiatrist takes responsibility for the decision to commit or to discharge, much of the screening and decision-making is done by other mental health workers; the decision to release a patient is often based on the opinions of aides and orderlies and "mental health technicians," although the hospital chart shows the signature of the physician. (A friend of mine has recently given me a definition of mental health technician for his state: "an orderly with an Associate of Arts degree [a two-year college course degree] or less.")

Only a very small percentage of the population is ever directly threatened with commitment, but everyone in society – except the most deranged and the most committable – understands that if you overstep certain lines the penalty may be either police power intervention or commitment – and sometimes both. We have tried to sweeten the commitment threat by insisting that as many patients as possible come into the hospitals as voluntary patients, but the iron hand is heavy in this velvet glove; the patient often signs in voluntarily only because the threat is that if he does not he will be committed involuntarily anyway and when the voluntary patient wants to leave the hospital he is informed he can be detained for a fixed number of days while the decision is made whether he should be committed involuntarily. We have the patient both coming and going.

Psychiatrists have many other kinds of authority, more kinds each year, but the power to commit is a basic underpinning of psychiatric authority; it sets psychiatrists apart from others in our society. The only other person in our society who has the power to deprive a noncriminal of his liberty is the juvenile court judge; when psychiatrists and juvenile court judges work together deciding on the question of detention or liberty for those subjected to their authority it is almost impossible to challenge their joint decisions.

The power to give an excuse for activities that would otherwise be considered criminal is also a great exercise of psychiatric authority. During the period from 1800 until the use of capital punishment was discontinued in the early 1960s, the psychiatrist who could testify that a defendant lacked criminal responsibility had a life-and-death power over that defendant. Of course the decision was not the psychiatrist's; it belonged to judge or jury; but the special expertise of the psychiatrist made it possible for judges and juries to comfort-

---

[12]See, for example: *Dixon v. Attorney General of Pennsylvania*, 325 F. Supp. 966 (M.D. Pa. 1971); *Lessard v. Schmidt*, 349 F. Supp. 1376 (E.D.Wis. 1974); *Suzuki v. Quisenberry*, 411 F. Supp. 1113 (D. Hawaii 1976); *Lynch v. Baxley*, 386 F. Supp. 378 (M.D. Ala. 1974); *Bell v. Wayne County General Hospital*, 384 F. Supp. 1085 (E.D. Mich . 1974).

ably decide that a defendant should or should not receive the extreme penalty. Today the death penalty is not a realistic threat but then neither is there the probability that once existed that a defendant not guilty by reason of insanity will spend the rest of his life in a mental hospital — sometimes the holdings of the criminally irresponsible are incredibly short — and lawyers are utilizing this kind of psychiatric expertise and authority increasingly when their trial tactics indicate it may be useful.[13]

Commitment and the involuntary treatment of mental patients, professional evaluations on culpability for crimes — these were the two areas where the authority of the psychiatrist was first brought into prominence. Then there were associated decision-making functions. By 1900 psychiatrists were also often used to testify about whether wills should be broken, whether contracts should be abrogated, whether guardians should be appointed.

The addition of Freudian concepts to the psychiatric armamentarium added enormously to its authority. In the first place, the concept of unconscious determinism carried with it the related concept that the psychiatrist was the person uniquely capable of understanding behavioral cause and effect. Secondly, the pre-Freudian psychiatrist dealt with the psychotically disturbed, but Freud made the neurotic and the character disorder subjects of psychiatric authority. Thirdly, the Freudian optimism about use of an abreactive and cathartic verbal process to induce change has given psychiatrists the status of promoters of change, rehabilitators; before Freud they were primarily custodians, caretakers. Our society emphasizes — rightly or wrongly — the efficacy of therapy; Philip Rieff has called his book *The Triumph of the Therapeutic: Uses of Faith after Freud.*[14] Fourth, unlike the pre-Freudian psychiatrist who was an expert only on abnormal mental states, the post-Freudian has developed theories of child-rearing, societal structuring, and so the present day psychiatrist has great authority as a kind of universal authority — who not only knows more than the rest of society about schizophrenia, and depression, and conversion symptoms, and hypochondriasis — but also about love and war, crime and punishment, morality and permissiveness and other profound aspects of life. Experts often disagree, and courts and the public both discount much of what psychiatrists say. Nevertheless, the Freudian grafting of medical psychology to the established neuropsychiatry led to a widespread acceptance that psychiatrists are experts about such larger issues.

With this extra authority, psychiatrists became involved in many aspects of the criminal justice system; in particular they advised judges on the disposition of sentenced offenders. They developed correctional rehabilitation programs that then became the justification for lengthened sentences because the goal of the sentence was no longer punishment but change and personal growth.

The Magnitude of Psychiatric Authority

Perhaps an academic forensic psychiatrist like myself (who rarely does evaluations for court purposes and so may perhaps be less biased in favor of psychi-

---

[13] See Jonas Robitscher and Roger Williams, "Should Psychiatrists Get Out of the Courtroom?" *Psychology Today* 11 (December 1977): 85.

[14] Philip Rieff, *The Triumph of the Therapeutic* (New York: Harper & Row, 1966).

atric infallibility than some less academic colleagues), made aware through clippings and case reports of the poignancy of some of the real-life situations where psychiatric determinations are so crucial, is in a particularly good position to become conscious of the magnitude of psychiatric authority.

One recent example is a New York City woman with two children who decided she needed attention for her emotional problems. She left the children (one aged seven years, the other aged six months) with a neighbor and went to Bellevue Hospital where she expected to receive outpatient care. Instead, she was admitted to the hospital and was there six days. The New York City Bureau of Child Welfare took custody of her children during this time without any authorization from her; after her discharge from the hospital she repeatedly demanded the return of her children but was denied this without any hearing or court order. The institution which took care of one of her children stated in its records that she was "sweet" but "not mother material." The children were authorized to be admitted to more permanent foster care instead of temporary emergency placement on the ground of "mental illness of the person caring for the child," although there had never been any official determination that the mother was mentally ill. The mother finally received legal help and 27 months after she had lost her children she filed a writ of habeas corpus petition; this was denied and she was found guilty of neglect; the alleged "neglect" then became the rationale for the legal loss of custody of the children. Three years later this finding was reversed on the ground that the mother had been denied the opportunity to present evidence rebutting the allegations of neglect. But the children still were not returned to her because the Family Court apparently desired to maintain the status quo pending a redetermination of the question of neglect.[15] Whether this lady was or was not a good or fit mother is not the question I wish to address; I merely want to point out the powerful effects of even such seemingly innocuous psychiatric decisions as the decision to hold for temporary observation or the characterization of a mother as "not mother material."

Let us try to get a grasp of the great number of ways in which psychiatrists can exercise their authority.

I have said commitment and criminal responsibility determinations are examples of the exercise of psychiatric authority; let me briefly go through a list of the number of other ways.

Psychiatrists determine financial competency; they decide when contracts may be abrogated, when guardians should be appointed.

They can deprive retarded or mentally disabled parents of their children, determine that some potential adoptive parents are not sufficiently stable to be parents, and in cases where there is no question of mental illness they can determine which of two parents will prevail in a custody dispute.

They can order retarded girls eugenically sterilized. Not infrequently in other countries, less frequently in the United States, they have had sexual offenders castrated to alter their behavior.

They exert enormous authority in the criminal justice and prison systems by

---

[15] *Duchesne v. Sugarman*, No. 76-7475 (2nd Cir., Sept. 28, 1977), *Clearinghouse Review*, Nov. 1977, 658.

their evaluations. Prison terms, prison assignments, recommendations for parole are all determined as the result of psychiatric and psychological evaluations.
Recently a psychologist described to a law school class the purposes for which
defendants were sent to his forensic services unit; they were sent, he said, to
determine competency to stand trial and criminal responsibility and also for
the evaluator's report on mitigating circumstances and for his dispositional recommendation.

They can divert people who are accused of some crimes from the criminal
justice system to the mental health system and hold them there forever.

They can find an accused not competent to stand trial and deprive him of
the chance to prove his innocence or enter objections to the way testimony
against him was gathered; until a Supreme Court decision of several years ago
they could retain the incompetent in a hospital for the criminally insane forever.[16]

They have great power over committed patients (and in most hospitals over
voluntary patients as well) to use restraints, force medication, force electroshock therapy, force behavior modification programs, to control all the aspects
of institutional living. Although the lobotomy has been phased out of existence,
in a period from the early 1940s until the early 1950s, some 50,000 lobotomies
were performed in the United States.[17] Had psychiatrists and neurosurgeons
not been restrained by the courts, they would now be doing more sophisticated
experimental psychosurgery on some involuntary patients to eliminate violence.[18]

They not only provide excuses for people accused of crimes but also for
many others — so that someone who fails in a job need not lose that job because he has a psychiatric reason for failure. One of the most significant ways,
Seymour Halleck has said, that psychiatry affects society is by excusing selected individuals from meeting ordinary social obligations.[19] (A psychologist recently wrote a University Academic Standing Committee and said, not unchar-
acteristically, that his patient should not be expelled from the university for
academic failure because the failure had been caused by the psychological phenomenon of fear of failure.)

Psychiatrists and other behavioral scientists can classify people on the basis
of testing, evaluations, diagnostic procedures, and profiling so that people are
categorized and then sent into various tracks and channels — institutional dispositions, educational tracks, vocational tracks. Behavioral scientists are widely
used in industry to make personnel decisions.

On the other hand, they can prevent people from securing jobs or force the

---

[16]*Jackson v. Indiana,* 406 U.S. 715 (1972).

[17]Peter R. Breggin, "The Return of Lobotomy and Psychosurgery," *Congressional Record* (Feb. 24, 1972): E1602–E1611.

[18]*Kaimowitz v. Department of Mental Health,* Civil No. 73–19, 434-AW (Cir. Ct. Wayne Co., Mich., July 10, 1973), reported in part in *Pris. L. Rep.* 2 (1973) 433 and 42 U.S.L.W. 2063 (1973). The court's opinion is reproduced in Alexander Brooks, *Law, Psychiatry and the Mental Health System* (Boston: Little, Brown, 1974), pp. 902–924.

[19]Seymour Halleck, "The Power of the Psychiatric Excuse," *Psychiatry Digest* 33 (March 1972): 35–44.

separation of people from their jobs on the finding of mental illness or disability or unsuitability. They can rule that some people are not dependable enough for security-sensitive jobs.

They can decide when someone should get early retirement and other benefits as a result of being ruled psychiatrically unfit to continue to work.

They assess psychic damage after accidents and other injuries including medical malpractice and give evidence that allows the personal injury lawyer to bring his case to court.

They can force people into psychiatric treatment under the threat of loss of job, loss of welfare benefits, revocation of parole, imposition of sentence, loss of custody of a child. Psychotherapy must then be entered into whether or not it is desired.

They can excuse a soldier from military duty and they were responsible for excusing thousands from Vietnam duty. They can determine which soldier should be separated from the service and the character — whether honorable or less than honorable — of their discharges.

Before abortions were made legal, they secured abortions for hundreds of thousands of women on the basis of an alleged "psychiatric need" and they will probably soon be used again to authorize federally-funded abortions for indigent mothers who without a finding of psychiatric need would not be entitled to a free abortion procedure.

They have been used to preserve order, particularly on college campuses and in prisons, through group therapy and anger-resolving techniques (although the anger may have been appropriate anger). In prisons and juvenile institutions they authorize nonmedical personnel to dispense and administer tranquilizers in order to preserve an atmosphere of decorum.[20]

Psychiatrists have also assumed authority over many conditions which were formerly not considered psychiatric and by redefining them as medical and psychiatric have brought them under coverage of medical insurance policies — marriage problems, other adjustment problems, antisocial behavior all can be considered psychiatric, and the authority of the psychiatrist decrees that when these problems are treated by a psychiatrist — or by someone acting under the authority of a psychiatrist (but not by an equally well-trained therapist not acting under the authority of a psychiatrist) — the expense shall be considered reimbursable. Thus a whole new contingent of prospective patients, not suffering from recognized psychiatric conditions but from what have been called "disorders of living," has come within the ambit of psychiatry.

Psychiatry deals with the individual specifically, but psychiatric authority is also used more broadly in ways that do not clearly imperil individual liberties but that set group and societal standards and help determine how we shall live, under what laws, and who shall govern us, and may in the long run, by changing our attitudes (concerning, for example, personal responsibility), have an even greater effect on the individual and his relation to society. When psychiatrists choose certain values in preference to others — the work ethic in preference to hedonism — or state that one behavior pattern is not preferable to another — as

---

[20] "Many Jailed Females Get Mood Drugs," *Atlanta Constitution*, (Aug. 8, 1977): 8-A.

they did in the case of homosexuality and heterosexuality[21] — they are setting
the norms for society. Many other changes in societal norms have been accomplished through psychiatric authority. By presenting "scientific" points-of-view
of the desirability of many aspects of modern living — on marriage, divorce, fi-
delity, premarital experimentation, the importance of the orgasm, the significance of perversions, the relative value of orgasms achieved through masturba-
tion and through intercourse, the roles of men and women and the relationship
of these roles, the value of permissive versus nonpermissive child rearing, the
usefulness and the appropriateness of various life styles — the psychiatrist helps
set the tone and enforce the structure (or weaken the structure) of society.

On a still more general level, psychiatrists make political pronouncements
about the psyciatric pathology of world leaders, have occasionally — rarely —
tried to influence our votes, propose methods to promote world peace. They
recommend large-scale societal reforms; they sometimes propose a massive restructuring of society as the answer to problems of mental malfunctioning.
Some psychiatrists have recently called racism the most serious psychiatric disease. Some psychiatrists have used their psychiatric authority to promote Marxism. Philip Lichtenberg asks whether psychoanalysis which is so often used to
enforce existing and prevailing values cannot and should not be used as a means
of promoting radical personal and social change.[22] *Issues in Radical Therapy*
asks whether therapy should not be used to promote growth and change rather
than conformity and the status quo.[23]

My point is not that all these psychiatric interventions are bad or represent
an excess of psychiatric authority. Some of them I think are ominous, but
many of the determinations made by psychiatrists need to be made by someone in society and I think psychiatrists if they are well informed and thoughtful and conscious of the effect of their authority are the proper people to make
them. Unlike Thomas Szasz, I do not see mental illness as a myth[24] and thus I
do not see all exercise of psychiatric authority as invalid; unlike Karl Menninger
I do not see the possibility of psychiatry withdrawing from involvement in
some of the more difficult phases of legal decision-making concerning mentally
disabled people.[25] My point is that psychiatrists have not stopped to consider
the extent of their power; they act in what they perceive to be the best interest
of the patient — like Sir William Bradshaw advising on when and when not to
have children, like Janet Gotkin's doctor trying to stamp out emotion with di-

---

[21] In December 1973, the Board of Trustees of the American Psychiatric Association adopted a text
prepared by Robert Spitzer legitimizing homosexuality; it eliminated homosexuality as a category of psychiatric disease and stated that homosexuality was "one form of sexual behavior" not by itself a psychiatric disorder and so not to be listed any longer in the official diagnostic manual.

[22] Philip Lichtenberg, *Psychoanalysis: Radical and Conservative* (New York: Springer Pub. Co., 1969).

[23] Some examples of advocacy of therapy for political change (among many others that have appeared
in *Issues in Radical Therapy*) are: Judy Henderson, "Emotions and the Left," *Issues in Radical Therapy*
18 (Spring 1977): 10—12; Terry Kupers, "Can Therapy be Radical?," *Issues in Radical Therapy* 20 (Fall
1977): 21—22; and Carl Boggs and William Caspary, "Therapy and Revolutionary Change," *Issues in Radical Therapy* 19 (Spring 1977): 4—6.

[24] Thomas Szasz, *The Myth of Mental Illness* (New York: Hoeber-Harper, 1961); Thomas Szasz, *Law,
Liberty, and Psychiatry* (New York: Macmillan, 1963).

[25] Karl Menninger, *The Crime of Punishment* (New York: Viking, 1968).

rection, interpretation, and chemotherapy — and they do not look at the totality of their interventions, the long-range effect on the patient, the effect on society.

Questioning the Use of Psychiatric Authority

The psychiatrist sitting in his office counselling and advising, occasionally in the past certifying an abortion, occasionally committing a patient, rarely getting involved in court testimony, not involved in institutional work, has proceeded happily on his course unmindful of the tremendous authority he and his fellow psychiatrists play in American life. When he talks about abuse of psychiatric authority one topic, and one topic alone, comes to his mind; he knows that Soviet psychiatrists have labeled political dissenters mentally ill on the basis of their political beliefs, and he deplores this. Through his union, the American Psychiatric Association, he passes resolutions against this practice[26] — and so he can now rest content that he is on the side of right concerning the misuse of psychiatric authority.

For many years there was almost no questioning of the use of psychiatric authority. Whatever opposition there was came from such reformers as Mrs. E. P. W. Packard and Dorothea Dix who believed, correctly, that Nineteenth Century America did not do enough to protect people from improper commitment, and from such journalists as Albert Deutsch who documented the poverty of the state hospital environment. Better commitment laws and better state hospitals appeared to be the answers to abuse of psychiatric authority.

For the most part, there was no recognition that psychiatry had a potential for abuse or had abused its authority. During most of this century the psychiatric literature contained pleas that society rely more on psychiatric authority, that psychiatrists be given more scope in commitment, a larger role in dealing with criminal defendants, new powers to deal with sexual offenders and defective delinquents and juvenile offenders, and that there be less legalistic protection for the patient in the civil commitment process. Before the problem of the too powerful or too intrusive behavioral scientist received much professional and scholarly attention, novelists and playwrights began to deal with this theme. I would date the responsible professional questioning of psychiatric authority to as recently as 1954. In a book entitled *Psychiatry and the Law*[27] a number of contributors called for a greater reliance on psychiatry in the criminal justice system, but there were some glimmerings on the part of three of the contributors that there were difficulties inherent in such dependence.

George Dession, Lines Professor of Law at Yale University, raised the question of the evaluating psychiatrist who interviews a patient and diagnoses him

---

[26] Starting in 1971, the American Psychiatric Association, the American Psychoanalytic Association, and the Royal College of Psychiatrists have passed resolutions condemning "the use of psychiatric facilities for the detention of persons solely on the basis of their political dissent." In 1977 the World Psychiatry Association Congress by a vote of 90—88 condemned the Soviet Union for "systematic abuse of psychiatry for political purposes in the USSR," *Atlanta Constitution* (Sept. 2, 1977): A-8.

[27] Paul Hoch and Joseph Zubin, eds., *Psychiatry and the Law* (New York: Gruene and Stratton, 1955) (Proceedings of the 43rd Annual Meeting of the American Psychoanalytical Association, New York, June 1953).

as a potentially dangerous and aggressive psychopathic sex offender although so far the individual has done nothing more serious than expose himself.[28] He pointed to the growing acceptance of sexual psychopath statutes and pointed out that such statutes represented an addition to the criminal justice system of preventive and welfare concepts which had previously been identified with health and mental health systems. In the same volume, Harold Lasswell discussed the influence of psychiatric opinion on legislative policy[29] and Lawrence Z. Freedman of the Yale Study Unit in Psychiatry and Law called attention to the value-laden orientation of psychiatry.[30]

In 1958 the first powerful voice of protest was raised about the growing power of psychiatrists in corrections. Michael Hakeem's "A Critique of the Psychiatric Approach to Crime and Corrections" considered some of the issues that Dession, Lasswell, and Freedman had raised, but Hakeem emphasized the real and current abuses instead of theoretical and potential abuses.[31] He quoted such leading psychiatrists of the period and such lawyers as Dr. Karl Menninger, Dr. Manfred Guttmacher, Dr. Benjamin Karpman, Justice William O. Douglas, Judge David Bazelon, and Abraham Fortas for the proposition that psychiatry should take a more commanding and authoritarian role in the approach to the problems of crime and the reform of corrections. Hakeem also cites a very few psychiatrists – Dr. Jerome Hall, Dr. Frederick Wertham, and Dr. Thomas Szasz – for their warnings that psychiatry was not as scientific as some of its practitioners claimed and that psychiatric authority was often used arbitrarily and harmfully.

Hakeem's article contains a unique collection of claims by psychiatrists for the efficacy of their methods and the reliability of their judgments. Modern psychiatrists would not make some of these statements not because they are necessarily less authoritarian or more civil liberties-oriented but because they are more sophisticated and they know the opposition, the derision such claims would raise. Hakeem quotes Karl Menninger: "The scientific attitude as shown in psychiatry must sooner or later completely displace existing legal methods" of dealing with criminality.[32]

Psychiatry took its biggest step toward self-criticism when in 1961 the monumental study of the American Bar Foundation, *The Mentally Disabled and the Law*, was published.[33] This collection of laws of all the United States jurisdictions made it possible to discuss forensic psychiatric topics without spending months in library research collecting basic data. The year 1961 also saw the appearance of Thomas Szasz's *The Myth of Mental Illness*[34] and Erving Goff-

---

[28] George Dession, "Deviation and Community Sanctions," in *Psychiatry and the Law, ibid.*, pp. 1–12.

[29] Harold Lasswell, "Legislative Policy, Conformity and Psychiatry," in *Psychiatry and the Law, ibid.*, pp. 13–40.

[30] Lawrence Z. Freedman, "Conformity and Nonconformity," in *Psychiatry and the Law, ibid.*, pp. 41–53.

[31] Michael Hakeem, "A Critique of the Psychiatric Approach to Crime and Correction," *Law and Contemporary Problems* 23 (1958): 650–682.

[32] *Ibid.*, p. 651.

[33] Samuel Brakel and Ronald Rock, eds., *The Mentally Disabled and the Law* (Chicago: Univ. of Chicago Press, 1971).

[34] Szasz, *supra*, note 24.

man's *Asylums.*[35] The publication the following year of Ken Kesey's brilliant *One Flew Over the Cuckoo's Nest*[36] particularly called the attention of the public to the extent of pscyiatric authority. Since then there has been an expanding literature attacking psychiatric authority on the ground that it lacks legitimacy (the position of Szasz, Leifer,[37] and Laing[38]) and that it is used to deny civil rights (Bruce Ennis,[39] Nicholas Kittrie,[40] Alan Dershowitz[41]).

Recent Changes

Certainly the public seeking help with emotional or mental problems — or merely with "problems of living" — has not been deterred from psychiatry by its critics. Bertram Brown, recently resigned Director of the National Institute of Mental Health, has said that in spite of the criticisms of psychiatry the demand for psychiatric services has shown no evidence of decline and he predicts that the demand will continue to grow for another decade.[42] Courts have greatly increased their requests for psychiatric consultations. Judges and juries, families, the police, correctional personnel, teachers, personnel officers more and more rely on psychiatric services.

The great change that has occurred is that courts have imposed limits on psychiatric authority but only in a few situations. Ever since the case of *Heryford v. Parker*[43] in 1968, we have had courts saying that the deprivation of liberty of a civil commitment can be experienced as painfully as a criminal punishment and should be given considerable procedural protections. Since that time some states by court decisions and others by acts of legislatures have tightened the standards of civil commitment. Some courts have gone so far as to give patients a right to remain silent during a commitment evaluation and not have that factor favoring commitment (analogous to a right against self-incrimination); they have required proof of committability far above civil court standards, sometimes requiring the "beyond a reasonable doubt" standard that we use for criminal convictions. Courts have prohibited psychiatrists from holding patients under disadvantageous conditions and have dictated the kind of treatment patients deserve; they have limited the power of psychiatrists to hold nondangerous committed patients; they have limited the power of psychiatrists to hold patients not competent to stand trial.[44] The development of a body of legal cases specifying the rights of patients — going so far as the right to refuse

---

[35] Erving Goffman, *Asylums* (Garden City, N.Y.: Anchor Books, 1961).

[36] Ken Kesey, *One Flew Over the Cuckoo's Nest* (New York: Viking Press, 1971). (Originally published 1962.)

[37] Ronald Leifer, *In the Name of Mental Health: The Social Functions of Psychiatry* (New York: Science House, 1969).

[38] R. D. Laing, *The Politics of Experience* (New York: Panteon Books, 1967).

[39] Bruce Ennis, *Prisoners of Psychiatry* (New York: Harcourt, Brace-Jovanovich, 1972).

[40] Nicholas Kittrie, *The Right to be Different* (Baltimore: Johns Hopkins Press, 1971).

[41] Alan Dershowitz, "The Psychiatrists's Power in Civil Commitment: A Knife that Cuts Both Ways." *Psychology Today* 3 (Feb. 1969): 42–44, 46–47.

[42] "Criticisms Haven't Reduced Psychiatric Service Demand," *Clinical Psychiatry News* (Aug. 3, 1975): 3.

[43] *Heryford v. Parker,* 396 F.2d 393 (10th Cir. 1968).

[44] See *supra*, note 16.

medication under some conditions[45] and the concomitant growth of a mental health bar have been the most effective limiting agents on the power of psychiatrists. But this kind of limitation of psychiatric authority is cumbersome, expensive, and it has aroused the antagonism of psychiatrists. More important, it only deals with a very few of the most flagrant abuses of psychiatric authority. Many of the items in our long list of the uses of psychiatry remain subject only to the psychiatrist's own self-regulation and self-control.

It is not only the patient who is committed under vague statutory criteria or the defective delinquent who serves a longer period in the hospital for the criminally insane than the maximum for his crime who has been abused by psychiatry. Many abuses of psychiatry go completely unregulated. One of the greatest abuses are the overreaching claims, as when Texas psychiatrists state they *know* that sociopathy is equated with impossibility of rehabilitation and so provide the testimony of continuing dangerousness that is necessary before the death sentence can be imposed,[46] or when the child psychiatrist on the basis of a one-hour evaluation *determines* that one parent is completely fit and one completely unfit to have custody of a child. In spite of the literature that has developed concerning the inadequacies of the psychiatric diagnostic classification and the fallibility of psychiatric predictions, psychiatrists continue to affect the lives of people by presenting their opinions as if they were truly scientific, by acting as if their data were harder than they were.

In spite of all the potential for abuse of authority, the average psychiatrist, who does not work in an institutional setting and who rarely commits patients, continues to be unmindful of this problem. Ask him about abuse of psychiatric authority and he will tell you about how Soviet psychiatrists force ideologies on political dissenters who have been labeled mental patients. Through his participating in the American Psychiatric Association, he helps pass resolutions deploring this practice – so he can rest content that he is doing his part to establish the proper limits of psychiatric authority.

Vladimir Bukovsky, himself a political patient in Russia for fifteen months and the author with Semyon Gluzman of the *Manual on Psychiatry for Dissidents,*[47] has estimated that at least 2,000 political dissidents are now being held in mental hospitals in the Soviet Union. The Soviet Union has twelve special psychiatric hospitals which are not under the Ministry of Health but are under the Ministry of Internal Affairs.[48] When Victor Fainberg was interviewed by his

---

[45] Three papers on the right to refuse treatment presented at the annual American Academy of Psychiatry and Law meeting in 1976 were published in *Bulletin of the American Academy of Psychiatry and the Law* 5, no. 1 (1977). These are Joseph Cocozza and Mary Elick, "The Right to Refuse Treatment: Administrative Considerations," pp. 8–14; and Kenneth Wing, "The Right to Refuse Treatment: Legal Issues," pp. 15–19. See also Marvin Stone, "The Right of the Psychiatric Patient to Refuse Treatment," *Journal of Psychiatry and Law* 4 (Winter 1976): 515–533.

[46] See George Dix, "The Death Penalty, 'Dangerousness,' Psychiatric Testimony and Professional Ethics," *Amer. Journal of Criminal Law* 5 (May 1977), 151–215.

[47] Vladimir Bukovsky and Semyon Gluzman, "A Manual on Psychiatry for Dissenters," *Survey* (Winter/Spring 1975): 176–198. (Reprinted by the Working Group on the Internment of Dissenters in Mental Hospitals, [London: 1976].)

[48] Peter Reddaway, "Psychiatric Prisoners," *Time,* (Feb. 28, 1972): E2; Clayton Yeo, "Psychiatry, the Law and Dissidents in the Soviet Union," *The Review* (International Commission of Jurists), nos. 12–15 (1974–75): 34–41, 38, 39; E. Fuller Torrey, "The Serbsky Treatment," *Psychology Today* 11 (June 1977): 38, 41–42.

psychiatrist and when he asked his psychiatrist why he was being held in a mental hospital, he was told his disease was dissent.[49] The Soviet Union is not the only country that uses psychiatry to enforce political ideology; Uruguay in recent years has used the same practice, and allegations have been made of political uses of psychiatry in Argentina, Chile, Czechoslovakia, and Rumania.[50]

But Americans can remember when youths arrested for participating in a racial demonstration to secure integration of a public swimming pool were sent for psychiatric evaluation, and the cases of Ezra Pound and General Edwin Walker, both held in psychiatric hospitals for political rather than medical reasons, are too well known to need further recounting. Until very recent years many individuals who chose to lead a different lifestyle — were promiscuous, used marijuana, were irresponsible — ran the risk of being labeled psychiatrically ill; drug users are still routinely sentenced to treatment programs. In very recent years we have had revelations about the use of CIA-employed psychiatrists in bizarre mind-control experiments and in the development of "profiles" on a Nixon political opponent.

The Role of the American Psychiatric Association

Very little action or policing or even self-criticism of psychiatry has come from psychiatry itself. In 1958 in his Presidential Address to the American Psychiatric Association, Harry Solomon said that after 114 years of effort only a few state hospitals had adequate staffs as measured against the minimum standards of the APA even though these standards were a compromise between what would really be adequate and "what it was thought had some possibility of being realized."[51] In the intervening years, the American Psychiatric Association has not devoted time or energy to this problem; it has waited for courts to force minimum staffing standards on hospitals. In 1960 Morton Birnbaum proposed that there was a constitutionally guaranteed right to a minimal standard of treatment for involuntary patients that should require state hospitals to bring the standards for hospital staff up to minimum requirements for private accredited hospitals;[52] the APA responded by abolishing the staffing ratios for private hospitals, and by passing a Council statement that "the definition of treatment and the appraisal of its adequacy are matters for medical determination."[53]

Except for forthright action to protect the rights of homosexuals[54] — based on the official APA policy that homosexuality does not necessarily represent psychopathology — the APA has not been concerned with actions to protect or improve the lot of most domestic mental patients. It has abdicated responsibili-

---

[49] Torrey, *ibid.,* p. 48.

[50] "Soviet Psychiatric Practices Criticized," *Science News* 112 (Sept. 10, 1977): 164–165.

[51] Harry Solomon, "Presidential Address," *Amer. Journal of Psychiatry* 115 (1958): 1–9, 7.

[52] Morton Birnbaum, "The Right to Treatment," *American Bar Assoc. Journal* 46 (1960): 499–505.

[53] American Psychiatric Association, *Standards for Psychiatric Facilities* (Washington, D.C.: APA, 1969), p. 29; American Psychiatric Assn., Official Actions," *Amer. Journal of Psychiatry* 123 (1967): 1458.

[54] American Psychiatric Association, "Official Actions: Position Statement on Homosexuality and Civil Rights," *Amer. Journal of Psychiatry* 131 (1974): 497. See also *supra,* note 21.

ty completely in the field of state hospital improvement. Confidentiality is a concern, but it is hard to know whether it is the interest of the patient or the doctor that has led to action on this subject. The Soviet Union's practices have been a concern; it is easier to be assertive about faraway problems than about problems at home.

One of the major ways to see that psychiatric authority is used more appropriately is to improve the conditions under which patients are held, and the APA has done remarkable little to see that psychiatrists, who are trained as the result of great expenditures of government funds, use some of their training for state hospital patients; or that inadequately trained foreign medical school graduates with poor language skills operating by virtue of special licenses not be given the major responsibility for state hospital patient care. Also, it has not been concerned that little or no psychiatric services are provided in most prison systems.

Now for the first time psychiatrists are beginning to find it necessary to study their relationship to society. Psychiatrists by temperament, a result of the selection process and the self-selection by which applicants are received into medical school and psychiatric residency programs, are happy in authoritarian roles. Most doctors are action-oriented and they are not philosophically inclined. They lack the intellectual rigor of lawyers in addressing these problems and they lack the compassion of humanists. But they are being dragged screaming into the twentieth century as the Anti-Authoritarian Century goes into its final quarter.

In 1972 when the issue of the use of psychiatry to control political dissidents in the Soviet Union was discussed by the Executive Committee of the American Psychiatric Association, the suggestion was made that psychiatry should also consider how it was used politically in all countries including the United States. An Ad Hoc Committee recommended a survey of how psychiatrists practice in United States institutions. The proposal was rejected by the APA Board of Trustees, leading one committee member, Judge David Bazelon, to say that "psychiatry is afraid to investigate itself."[55] Five years later the subject was finally considered in a meeting sponsored jointly by the APA and the Hastings Center (The Institute of Society, Ethics and the Life Sciences). Judd Marmor, former President of the APA, opened the meeting by referring to Bazelon's 1972 statement but denying its validity. "We weren't afraid," he said. "We knew abuse existed." And he ticked off a list of conflict of values problems in psychiatry: Is psychiatry an agent of social control? How is mental health defined? How do psychiatrists know that the unconscious motivations they ascribe to others do not affect their own diagnoses and prescriptions? Marmor did not explain why, if psychiatry was not afraid and knew that abuse existed, it had taken so long to begin to address the matter. Later in the same meeting Alan Stone quoted sociologist Eliot Freidson on professional etiquette: "There is concern among doctors about hiding abuse [that] is more powerful than their canons of ethics." Robert Michels recommended that psychiatrists redefine the therapeutic contract which now is ambiguous and encourages doctors to serve two masters.[56]

---

[55] Margaret McDonald, "Psychiatry: A Self Assessment," *Psychiatric News* (July 1, 1977): 1.
[56] *Ibid.*

The President of the Canadian Psychiatric Association in 1975 said, "on the whole, it is extraordinary how little attention has been paid to the formulation of a detailed code of psychiatric ethics on the one hand, or a philosophy of the morality of the whole treatment enterprise on the other."[57]

Other Possibilities for Change

If we cannot look to the APA for effective ways of dealing with the formulation of the role of psychiatry, are there other possibilities?

In 1972 I delivered a paper at the meeting of the American College of Legal Medicine in which I said that Legal Psychiatry requires more teaching time and more teaching skills, that it is the natural place in the medical school, psychiatric residency program and law school curriculum to consider "the social role of the psychiatrist, the delegation of power to the psychiatrists that formerly belonged to courts and administrative agencies, and the possible use and abuse of the formidable power that belongs to the modern psychiatrist."

I suggested a broader title than Legal Psychiatry to denote that role that Legal Psychiatry could play — Social Legal Psychiatry was the term I used — and I talked about this as the logical place in the curriculum to bring different interdisciplinary skills to bear — psychiatry, psychology, law, sociology, political science. Most of the paper was a discussion of how Legal Psychiatry could be taught more fully and more effectively.[58] The *American Journal of Psychiatry* turned down the paper; the anonymous reviewer gave as one reason the awkwardness of the term Social Legal Psychiatry. "It invites retort," he said, "Do you mean as opposed to antisocial illegal psychiatry?" I still feel that the medical school and psychiatric residency program curricula are the places where much more attention should be brought to bear on the problems of delineating the use of psychiatric authority. Since 1972, law schools have increased their interest in this field, and legal activism has accomplished a great deal as I have indicated, but the pressure of legal activism in curbing the authority of psychiatrists is not the equivalent of psychiatrists working out their own answers.

Psychiatrists and perhaps in particular psychiatric residents show no great interest in defining and curbing their power. The selection process which brings people into medical school and into psychiatric residency programs works against more humanistically and more socially conscious students; the intense competition and the emphasis on science as an undergraduate major that characterize admission to American medical schools act to favor students who are narrowly scientific, mechanistic, and materialistic in both the philosophic and economic senses of the word. Some psychiatrists are a notable exception, but it is striking how many more law students than psychiatric residents are interested in learning about the Right to Treatment or the Right to Refuse Treatment.

Ten years ago John Medelman, who had flunked out of medical school in his sophomore year, wrote an article for *Harper's* entitled "Why I am Not a Psychi-

---

[57] Dorothy Trainor, "CPA President Urges Greater Social, Ethical Consciousness," *Psychiatric News* (Nov. 5, 1975): 1.

[58] Jonas Robitscher, "The Changing Face of Legal Psychiatry: Or Social Legal Psychiatry" (Delivered at the Annual Meeting of the American College of Legal Medicine, Miami, Fla., May 13, 1972).

atrist."[59] Medelman described a long-time interest in psychiatry, his work in a mental hospital which in spite of its disillusioning aspects convinced him that psychiatry was his mission. But he found the preclinical years of medical school very unsatisfying and he did not do well. He wrote:

> We spent hundreds of hours with the struts and pulleys of the dead, hours the prospective psychiatrist should spend with the concepts and troubles of the living.

In some dim utopian future, Medelman predicts, psychiatric residents "might hear lectures by lawyers as well as doctors, and observe the seedy unhappiness of a courtroom instead of memorizing the muscles of the foot; they might hear about the monetary problems of state mental hospitals instead of trying to find whether they have pentose or fructose in their test tubes; and they might exchange lectures on tumor pathology for lectures on social anthropology and theories of ethics."

But the trend is in the other direction. Psychiatry is becoming more biologically-oriented, and as it continues to expand its influence and deal with more and more people it relies increasingly on quick interventions — crisis-oriented therapy, chemotherapy, behavior modification, and social work restructuring — to deal with patients' ills. The psychologically-minded dynamic therapist is more and more being displaced by a more manipulative kind of psychiatrist who does not want to deal with such psychiatric concepts as the unconscious, the transference, the countertransference, and working through to produce change but who nonetheless has inherited the authority and mystique which Freud has given to psychiatry. Lee Weiss has commented on this phenomenon:

> A cursory examination of the leading psychiatric journals will clearly indicate this trend. Articles on possible biological correlates of mental illness, somatic interventions, and descriptive diagnosis can be found in abundance. Psychiatric research is predominantly aimed at elucidating presumed biochemical abnormalities . . . or comparing the therapeutic efficacy of various somatic treatments. Psychiatric education has been moving in a similar direction, with much more emphasis on the biological substrata of abnormal behavior, descriptive diagnosis, and somatic treatment.

One of his conclusions is that the "current trend in training which emphasizes processes at the biological level at the expense of attention to other levels of analysis (behavior, intrapsychic social, etc.) . . . can only produce poorly educated psychiatrists unable to formulate cases in a comprehensive fashion or to utilize information from neighboring disciplines."[60] Along similar lines, Seymour Halleck has recently written that the increased emphasis on medical training in the postmedical school education of a psychiatrist is not likely to enhance the psychiatrist's functioning as a doctor to the mentally ill and may re-

---

[59] John Medelman, "Why I am Not a Psychiatrist," *Harper's* (Feb. 1967): 46–49.
[60] Lee Weiss, "The Resurgence of Biological Psychiatry: New Promise or False Hope for a Troubled Profession," *Perspectives in Biology and Medicine* 20 (Summer 1977): 573–585.

tard this capacity to learn many of the skills which are needed for effective psychiatric practice.[61]

But the medical model increasingly dominates psychiatry, and the psychologically-oriented are outnumbered by more biologically-oriented residents.

The hope that establishment psychiatry or new, younger psychiatrists will turn an appreciable amount of attention to the abuses of psychiatry seems nebulous. To the extent that continuing education can focus on these problems, it could be a help — but we know from experience that psychiatrists avoid nonclinical learning experiences; they will attend a meeting on confidentiality if they are in California and feel threatened by a court decision that may impair the confidentiality of the psychiatrist-patient relationship; they will not attend a meeting on the inequities of sexual psychopath legislation or the lack of psychiatric care in prisons.

Principles for Discussion

There is the need for the setting of limits — more limits than these external forces can provide. And we will have to be much more precise in deciding where these limits should be. We will have to rely on pressures from activist lawyers, courts, sociologists, the press, and an increasingly enlightened public to help psychiatrists stay within bounds. I cannot go too deeply into the specifics of these limits — the subject is too huge and too controversial — but I would like to throw out some principles that seem to me to be useful and in any case can provide a basis for discussion.

Psychiatrists should not have the authority of medicine in areas where their expertise is not medical or even scientific; for example, claims that they can use therapy to clear up problems of criminal deviancy should be exposed as overreaching.

It follows that the possibility of receiving therapy in an institutional setting should not be the rationalization for a detention longer than an appropriate purely punitive and deterrent detention. Indefinite or indeterminate holdings dependent on the certification of the psychiatrist that an individual diverted from the criminal justice system is "recovered," "cured," or "safe to be returned to society" should never be allowed; psychiatrists should be allowed to retain individuals only as long as they meet criteria for civil committability; if longer detentions are needed they should be labeled as punitive, which they are, and they should be protected by procedural safeguards.

Psychiatrists should decide where their primary loyalty lies — to the hospital for the criminally insane (or another state agency which pays their salaries) or to the ostensible "patient"; the patient should at all times understand that the doctor is not "his doctor" if the doctor has a higher loyalty to his employer.

Psychiatry should not be allowed to operate in an atmosphere of low visibility if there are coercive elements in the doctor-patient relationship. Use of pretrial reports and posttrial dispositional recommendation should be considered

---

[61] Seymour Halleck, "The Medical Model and Psychiatric Training," *Amer. Journal of Psychotherapy*. 30 (1976): 218–235.

suspect when they give the psychiatrist power which cannot be challenged through the adversary process.

The adversary system should be encouraged; use of impartial psychiatric experts and so-called "super experts" (specially trained or specially qualified legal psychiatric experts) should be suspect because their evaluations and recommendations carry too much weight and are not easily subject to challenge.

Pretrial diversion methods should be subject to rigid scrutiny, and other kinds of coercive therapy should also be considered potentially dangerous. The practice of sentencing well-to-do defendants to "psychiatric probation" should be considered suspect, since it discriminates against poor defendants and it often leads to a peculiar kind of therapy in which the patient cannot express himself for fear of its effect on the probation reports his therapist writes. (Just as the sinner formerly could purchase indulgences, the modern-day malfeasant who pays his weekly fee to his psychiatrist can win a favorable report.)

When psychiatric reports are used for important decisions — which parent should have custody of a child or whether a defendant is dangerous and needs a prolonged holding — the basis of the evaluation should be spelled out clearly; too many such reports are done hurriedly by inadequately trained psychiatrists who put only conclusions in their reports ("this man is a sociopath") and not the basis of the conclusions.

Procedural safeguards — such as the writ of habeas corpus — should be emphasized by courts; courts should stop relying on superficial indications of appropriate administration determinations to deny a patient his chance for a full-scale review. In spite of the psychiatrist's antipathy to procedural safeguards, they are necessary to keep psychiatrists from assuming too much authority.

When evidence of wrongdoing by psychiatrists is unearthed, (for example, the recent stories of Central Intelligence Agency employment of psychiatrists to plan improper experiments) the offending psychiatrists should be publicly identified, and they should be prosecuted when this is appropriate and in any event should be professionally disciplined. Professional discipline and license revocation should also be applied to psychiatrists who victimize their private patients.

Some central professional authority representing private practice as well as institutionally-employed physicians should be responsible for eliminating such long-standing abuses as use of irregularly licensed psychiatrists in state hospitals, deficiences of manpower in these institutions, and lack of psychiatric care and aftercare for prisoners.

The psychiatric excuse should not be allowed to operate unequally, such as excusing some students for failing examinations on the ground they are depressed thus giving them an advantage over other students or allowing some draft-eligible men to avoid military duty (as they did during the Vietnam conflict) on psychiatric certification while less advantaged men with similar pathology are forced to serve in their stead.

Patients should have actual — not theoretical — ability to secure legal help, have access to independent psychiatric expertise, and they should always be fully apprised of their legal rights.

It goes without saying that political ideologies should not be enforced by psychiatrists, but although it is easy to identify a blatant ideological bias, there are subtle ideologies and value systems which need to be clarified.

These are suggestions on some limits. You will have additional limits in mind.

Psychiatric authority continues to grow, few psychiatrists are willing to come to terms with the issue of the limits of psychiatric authority, and although courts and other external forces have indicated some of the boundaries beyond which psychiatrists cannot go, only the most rudimentary beginnings have been made in the consideration of this issue. This is an appropriate time — there will never be a better time — to think about and to set limits for the exercise of authority over those people who because they are designated patients are not entirely free — and sometimes not free at all — in a society that emphasizes freedom.

Comments on Robitscher's "The Limits of Psychiatric Authority"

Commentator: David Bakan*

Professor Robitscher's criticism of the psychiatric profession is sharp and scathing. Our world no longer allows itself to be taken in by mystiques. There is also an accelerated growth of human sensitivity to social injustice. Professor Robitscher's criticisms reflect both of these characteristics of the contemporary world. His criticisms must be taken to heart by the psychiatric profession and the community at large.

I find myself in virtually complete agreement with him in his criticisms. The arrogation of power by psychiatrists is much more than is warranted by circumstances. The limited amount of reliable, valid and accepted knowledge available to them hardly warrants the great social powers that they have. The methods for the selection, training and employment of psychiatrists are not distinguished; and often work to counter their intended functions. Rarely is there adequate provision for the proper review of important psychiatric decisions. Often the effects of psychiatric decisions are totally irreversible. Often what is intended to be benign turns out malignantly.

It seems to me that the disorder which is manifested in the various abuses that Robitscher has enumerated is very profound. It lies deep in the tissues of the total society. In probing the issues it is important that we do not content ourselves with blaming individual psychiatrists or the psychiatric profession as a whole. For culpability is characteristically the most superficial aspect of any social problem.

Let us have a quick glance at history. At about the same time as the great burst of urbanization and industrialization took place in the world, a new spirit took over in connection with jurisprudence in the 19th and 20th centuries. Instead of continuing to pursue what had sometimes become a relentless Gilbert and Sullivan-like "let the punishment fit the crime" approach, the courts openly assumed the responsibility of making their judgments in accordance with the *future,* in accordance with projected effects of their judgments on the society as a whole. The principle of specific culpability notwithstanding, the courts allowed decisions to be made on the basis of a variety of pieces of information concerning the person, the person's character, and the guessed future behavior of the person. An extreme manifestation of this frame of mind was in connection with the treatment of juveniles, in which the court had little obligation to even consider the offense, as such, with any seriousness at all; in which the critical judgment was whether the young person was or was not "delinquent."

The kind of program implicit in this approach called for a great increase in resources available to the courts. The program called for a giant step in research,

*Professor of Psychology, York University, Downsview, Ontario, Canada.

investigatory resources and a major supervisory role of the court in connection with the *character of people* as contrasted with simpler judgments of fact and law. Implicit in this new program also was a vast increase in government intrusion into the most intimate aspects of the lives of people. The public, I believe, never fully could participate in this changed program of the courts, and the resources that the program called for were never forthcoming from the public treasury. As a consequence, the courts have lived in a kind of in-between land of seemingly good intentions, on the one hand, and a condition of impotence with respect to the carrying out of the intentions, on the other. Thus, with some very few exceptions, to this very day the courts have very few real options except the option to punish or refrain; with some few options with respect to the nature of the punishment, limited choice of institutions, a shabby probation apparatus, or the like. The fact is that resources for quality alternatives at the court's disposal have always been scanty.

It is this historical situation which has made the profession of psychiatry important. The psychiatric profession largely owes its very existence to this situation. It is to be recalled that the original psychiatric profession of the 19th century was made up of the managers of the insane asylums, with the modern American Psychiatric Association having been originally, before changing its name, the association of the superintendents of these insane asylums.

At the very least, the historical M'Naughten rule (1843) allowed the court to make a decision regarding insanity on the basis of judicial judgment. For although it allowed for mental disease, it at least indicated what mental disease was in a way that a judge or jury might be qualified to decide: that at the time of committing the act, the party accused was laboring under such defect of reason, from disease of mind, as not to know the nature and quality of the act he was doing; or if he did know it, that he did not know that what he was doing was wrong.

However, *Durham v. United States* (1954) made it virtually necessary for the courts to seek the help of professionals. Or, perhaps the growing condition led to the delegation of judicial power to psychiatry implicit in *Durham v. United States*. In that decision a new test was explicated: that an accused is not criminally responsible if his unlawful act was the product of mental disease or mental defect. Aside from all of the vicissitudes associated with acceptance of such a rule, the fact is that courts have tended more and more to lean on the judgments of psychiatrists, under the assumption that in this way they carry out their duties with greater responsibility.

Professor Robitscher is quite right: There is virtually no visibility of the work of the psychiatrist. Few people know what happens in his office, in his mind, in the mental hospital, or even what the body of knowledge is that he is presumed to be the master of.

In a certain sense, invoking the name and image of Freud is a disservice and an untruth. For psychoanalysis, in which the psychoanalyst devotes hundreds or thousands of hours of uninterrupted attention to a single person, is one of the rarest of psychiatric activities. Most psychiatric contacts, particularly when the law is involved, are infinitely shabbier.

Most of the psychiatric contacts relevant to this discussion are with the indigent and variously disabled, involving payment to the psychiatrist for his services by a third party institution, and very often an institution associated with government. The structure of obligation is that the psychiatrist is responsible to a third party, and not to the person receiving the professional attention. And, unfortunately, a good deal of what passes as psychiatric attention constitutes a public intrusion into regions of personality and regions of private life, which have historically always been separated from the public sphere.

My reading of Professor Robitscher's paper produced a major thought which I would like to share with you as my final observation: The psychiatrist is something like a coroner; and perhaps that should be officially recognized and appropriately constituted. Let us consider the social role of the coroner. His main duty is to investigate cases of death where there is the possibility of some unnatural cause. The word coroner is derived from *corona,* meaning crown, and suggests the prior responsibility of the coroner to the state.

In a certain sense the coroner is not a professional. Professional usually connotes a primary responsibility to the client receiving professional services. The professional character of a physician inheres in the fact that he assumes a primary responsibility to the sick person, and a secondary responsibility to all others including himself. The same may be said of the professional character of the lawyer.

Now it is true that the coroner is often a physician by training. The knowledge and skill that he brings to bear is precisely the same as one would need for healing people. But the coroner has little interest in healing his "client." His pathology lab may be similar to any pathology lab. His examination of bodies may even be more thorough than that by physicians. But he has no interest in healing. His principal responsibility is to the state, and not to the interest of the person who is the focus of his investigation. And he receives his remuneration from a third party.

This comparison would be amusing if there were less cogency to it. The various observations of Professor Robitscher would suggest that perhaps the comparison is more cogent than, I am sure, some would want to believe.

It may well be that there is a need for an office analogous to that of the coroner, where the central interest is in the psychological characteristics of persons who come to the attention of the courts. If that be the case, it should be fully recognized and properly executed, with proper respect to due process. It seems to me that this is the logical conclusion that one must reach from Professor Robitscher's observations. There should be a separation of psychological assessment for the purpose of making legal decisions from assessment for treatment purposes. If there is need for professional services to the client, there must be guarantees that the interests of the client are primary in the relationship with the professional.

Indeed, if there is a single lesson which might be extracted from the work of Freud about the causes of mental disease, it is in the identification of punitive-type and judicial-type experiences in the life of the person as causes of such disease. Therapy can take place properly only in an atmosphere which is free of threat. Therefore, unless the judical functions and the therapeutic functions are relentlessly separated, there is little hope that the aims of the individual or the community can be realized through these mechanisms.

Comments on Robitscher's "The Limits of Psychiatric Authority"

Commentator: R. E. Turner*

The Psychiatrist as Physician

Without denying Professor Robitscher's point pertaining to the "authority of all those who make psychiatric decisions . . . practitioners who are not formal psychiatrists," I contend that we may not yet be ready to expand from individual disciplines in " . . . a field which is [indeed so] large [and] amorphous." Our society has, through its statutes, granted considerable authority to physicians. It is the psychiatrist as physician who holds authority most similar to that of his medical colleagues. In whatever problems and conditions in which psychiatrists become involved beyond the " . . . seriously abnormal mental states" — and whatever therapeutic approaches the psychiatrist undertakes, the psychiatrist remains a physician. We must remind ourselves that no physician can practice responsibly without a contingent of other professionals and technicians. We may argue that psychiatrists, in their decision-making role, are even more dependent on others, but is this actually so if we examine the input a physician seeks and receives in the general hospital?

Having said this, one must address oneself to the problem of the psychiatrist and the medical model. "Psychiatry is becoming more biologically oriented . . ." How does this affect the authority of the psychiatrist? Osmond of Princeton[1] developed a compilation of conceptual models of approaches to psychiatric illness. Jones of Dalhousie[2] said:

> If medicine is to maintain its rightful place in the human sciences, we must broaden our concepts of the cause of illness and develop more and more comprehensive approaches to prevention and therapy. Psychiatry has felt the need to examine and rethink its operational model earlier than general medicine . . . For the Greek Hippocrates everything in the ecology played a part in man's health and man's health was part of that ecological system. Jaeger, commenting on Hippocrates' volume — " . . . He, that is Hippocrates, does not isolate a disease and examine it as a special problem in itself. He looks steadily and clearly at the man who has the disease and sees him in all his natural surroundings, with their universal laws and their own special characteristics. . . . " The sicknesses of the 1970's result from multiple fac-

*M.D., F.R.C.P. (C) Professor of Forensic Psychiatry, University of Toronto, Canada.

[1] H. Osmond, "The Medical Model — Love It or Leave It," Tenth Annual Dinner, Sibley Memorial Hospital, Washington, D.C., reported in *Psychiatric News*, October 20, 1971. His models are moral, social, psychoanalytic, family interaction, conspiratorial, psychedelic, impaired, and medical.

[2] R. O. Jones, "Psychiatry, Medicine and the 1970's," Royal College Lecture, *Annals Royal College of Physicians and Surgeons of Canada*, April 1972.

tors: genetic, microbial, social, cultural, psychological, to name but a few. In much of current disease the specific medical model has little to offer — it must be supplemented by broader based models taking into account social, psychological and cultural factors, that is, the ecological model of Hippocratic medicine . . . this broader model will often identify basic factors in the production of human illness which demand change. Physicians are most strategically placed to identify and evaluate these and provide leadership in change."

And so is the psychiatrist — strategically placed to identify and evaluate authority and to provide leadership in change — from the base that Professor Robitscher has provided.

But we cannot leave this matter without attending to the problem of defining psychiatry, mental disorder, and psychiatrist which Professor Robitscher raised in his paper.

I would like to recommend three papers. The first, "Psychiatry Ltd." by D. Curran,[3] focusses on the dilemmas of ranging from demonstratable pathological lesions to every type of maladjustment. "In conclusion," he states, "when one looks at the vast fields that are unquestionably in the domain of psychiatry, and at how much still remains to be done, is it necessary, is it wise and may it not be rather premature to look for fresh fields to conquer or to fail in?" In the second, Emmanuel of Montreal puts a similar question in his article "Has Psychiatry Been Oversold?"[4] And Lewis suggests, in "Between Guesswork and Certainty in Psychiatry,"[5] that "there are occasions when a review of important areas of ignorance and doubt, and of the reasons for them, seems appropriate. Clearly we are a long way from certainty. . . . " We dare not ignore such notes of caution when examining the limits of psychiatric authority. It will not escape your notice that these three references are all from 1953–1957, i.e. the decade of lithium, reserpine, chlorpromazine, iproniozid, tricyclic anti-depressants and chlordiazepoxide — the advent of the chemotherapy period.

One further comment should be made. Robitscher's paper seems to polarize between "committal to mental hospitals" psychiatry, and psychiatry for the "well-functioning neurotic." What of the substantial number of patients seen in in-patient and out-patient psychiatric units of general hospitals and what is the authority of the psychiatrist in those settings?[6] Is the dichotomy of authority as applicable in the general hospitals? What of implicit and explicit authority? Does the general hospital psychiatric unit provide us with an intermediate model in which one can address the problems of authority?

Legislative and Governmental Authority

This is the area where the greatest ferment is taking place. As Robitscher remarks, "better commitment laws and better state hospitals appeared to be the

---

[3] D. Curran, "Psychiatry Ltd.," Special Article, *Canad. Psychiat. Assoc. J.* 68 (1953): 63–66.

[4] E. Emmanuel, "Has Psychiatry Been Oversold?" *Canad. Psychiat. Assoc. J.* 74 (1956): 259–262.

[5] A. Lewis, "Between Guesswork and Certainty in Psychiatry," 1957 Bradshaw Lecture, *Lancet,* Jan. 25, Febr. 1, 1958.

[6] In Ontario, there are 4,500 beds in psychiatric hospitals; 2,600 in some 54 general hospitals, for a population of 8,417,000.

answers to abuse of psychiatric authority." This is still true. It is the provincial or state legislatures by way of statutes that establish authority, and governments that provide the means by which the psychiatric task can be fulfilled.

Much has been said of "dangerousness" and commitment laws, and more is to come. Most Canadian provincial mental health statutes use the concept of "safety," e.g., in Ontario, the involuntary patient is "any person who, (a) suffers from mental disorder of a nature or degree so as to require hospitalization in the interests of his own safety or the safety of others; and (b) is not suitable for admission as an informal patient." The physician's application for involuntary admission must note facts indicating mental disorder he observes, other facts communicated by others to him, and he must state reasons why the person is not suitable for admission as an informal patient.

One could have spent this entire symposium on a discussion of mental health legislation. Further discussion in our respective countries should be mindful of Stone's "Mental Health and Law: A System in Transition"[7] as a companion to Professor Robitscher's paper.

Likewise, the 1955 paper, "Psychiatry and the Law" by Hoch and Zubin,[8] was referred to by Professor Robitscher as the date when "responsible professional questioning of psychiatric authority" really began. Future legal and psychiatric historians will undoubtedly comment that the advent decade of chemotherapy coincided with both caution about psychiatry being "oversold" or "Ltd." and the questioning of psychiatric authority.

In regard to legislative authority, I would like to commend "Paper Victories and Hard Realities"[9] — selected papers on the U.S. Supreme Court Decision, *O'Connor* v. *Donaldson.* It was the hope of that seminar that this publication be used as a guide for legislators. I will not refer to the decision itself except to say that *O'Connor* v. *Donaldson* poses an enigma. The issues of right to liberty, dangerousness, custodial care, capability of surviving safely and right to treatment are clearly stated. What I wish to emphasize here is the observation in the decision that " . . . the courts have ordered state governments to make extensive and expensive changes in facilities to ensure that patients are provided with appropriate treatment." As Professor Robitscher said, "one of the major ways to see that psychiatric authority is used more appropriately is to improve the conditions under which patients are held." The chapters by Bloom and Lottman in *Paper Victories* underline the fiscal dilemma and hard realities. Do states and provinces have the financial resources to comply with judicial rulings?

Judicial Authority

There is little case law in Canada on psychiatric authority or current provincial mental health legislation. Has there been a Canadian judicial interpretation relating to committal procedures?

---

[7] A. A. Stone, *Mental Health and Law: A System in Transition* (Rockville Maryland: National Institute of Mental Health, 1975).

[8] P. H. Hoch and J. Zubin, *Psychiatry and the Law* (New York: Grune and Stratton, 1955).

[9] V. Bradley and G. Clarke, eds., *Paper Victories and Hard Realities: The Implementation of the Legal and Constitutional Rights of the Mentally Disabled* (Washington, D.C.: The Health Policy Center, Georgetown University, 1976).

There are a few Canadian cases, e.g. *R. v. Fegan*, a bail review by Mr. Justice Lerner in the Supreme Court of Ontario, October 1977, concerning an application by the Crown for a detention order, and power in the court to remand to a psychiatric facility for a mental examination and assessment. This question involved both the Criminal Code of Canada, the Mental Health Act of Ontario and the Canadian Bill of Rights, 1960. Both detention and remand were upheld. The judgment referred to another Ontario Supreme Court case *Ex Parte Branco*, an application for habeas corpus before Mr. Justice Addy, which held that " . . . the examination is not a proceeding against the accused but, on the contrary, a proceeding conceived and given a statutory basis for the protection and benefit of the accused." Note the language in this decision.

R. v. Sweeney in the Ontario Court of Appeal, a decision written by Mr. Justice Zuber in March 1977, upheld the ruling that evidence was admissable that the appellant refused to submit to an examination by a psychiatrist and a psychologist retained by the Crown. As for the all important issue of criminal responsibility — the criminal law and the defense of insanity — the case of *R. v. Simpson*, January 1977, before the Ontario Court of Appeal, written by Mr. Justice Martin, updated the interpretation of Section 16 of the Criminal Code of Canada especially with regard to the concept of "disease of the mind."

This section of my commentary would be quite incomplete without reference to Professor Robitscher's hope for a more intensive and extensive dialogue about law and psychiatry with law students and psychiatric residents, lawyers and psychiatrists, practitioners, prosecutors, and the judiciary. Such a dialogue would involve specific cases, case law and statutes, clinical examples, etc. But the dialogue should, in addition, be within the framework of the writings of Hart,[10,11] Cardozo,[12] Horowitz,[13] Dworkin,[14] Lloyd[15] — to name but a few.

Accountability

As limits of psychiatric authority expand, psychiatry becomes even more involved in the many areas enumerated by Professor Robitscher, and as the list of therapeutic approaches grows, the greater becomes the need for mechanisms of accountability. This is a reason why I have focussed on the psychiatrist as physician. Systems of accountability are already in place — health discipline acts (e.g., a statutory list of professional misconduct in regulations), public hospitals acts, provincial or state colleges of physicians and surgeons (complaints and discipline committees) as well as medical record audit and hospital accreditation procedures. Provincial mental health legislation provides review boards for those held under a warrant of the lieutenant-governor (those unfit to stand trial or not guilty by reason of insanity). In addition, there is recourse to the courts,

---

[10] H. L. A. Hart, *Law, Liberty and Morality* (Stanford: Stanford University Press, 1963).
[11] H. L. A. Hart, *Punishment and Responsibility: Essays in the Philosophy of Law* (Oxford: Clarendon Press, 1968).
[12] B. N. Cardozo, *The Nature of the Judicial Process* (New Haven: Yale University Press, 1921).
[13] D. L. Horowitz, *The Courts and Social Policy* (Washington, D.C.: The Brookings Institution, 1977).
[14] R. Dworkin, *Taking Rights Seriously* (Cambridge Mass.: Harvard University Press, 1977).
[15] D. Lloyd, *The Idea of Law* (Harmondsworth: Penguin Books, A Pelican Original, 1964).

although as stated earlier, this has been used less frequently in Canada than the United States. There are some procedural safeguards. Are they sufficient to scrutinize psychiatric authority?

Ethics

Yet another reason for my reference to the psychiatrist as physician is to highlight the centuries-long ethical base from which we practice — from Hippocrates through Percival to the Codes of Ethics of both the American and Canadian Medical Associations.

You will recall the Official Actions section of the *American Journal of Psychiatry*[16] on "The Principles of Medical Ethics with Annotations Especially Applicable to Psychiatry." The Board of Directors of the Canadian Psychiatric Association has adopted in principle a commentary for psychiatrists on the Code of Ethics of the Canadian Medical Association compiled by Dr. Mellor of St. John's, Newfoundland, with annotations for psychiatrists enlarging on the physicians' code. Redlich and Mollica have written an "Overview: Ethical Issues in Contemporary Psychiatry."[17] And, as a source book, we now have available *Ethics in Medicine* edited by Reiser, Dyck and Curran.[18] The ethical aspects of psychiatry were considered to be of such importance at the VI World Congress of Psychiatry, Honolulu, 1977, that a plenary session was devoted to the subject.

Freedman of New York spoke of "A Question of Allegiance";[19] Chalke of Ottawa[20] about the psychiatric care of prisoners (about which he asked whether the Declaration of Hawaii was sufficient for the ethics relating to forensic

---

[16] *Am. J. Psychiat.* 130: 9 (September 1973).

[17] F. Redlich and R. F. Mollica, "Overview: Ethical Issues in Contemporary Psychiatry," *Am. J. Psychiat.* 133: 2 (Feb. 1976): 125–136.

[18] S. J. Reiser, A. J. Dyck, and W. J. Curran, *Ethics in Medicine: Historical Perspectives and Contemporary Concerns* (Cambridge, Mass.: The MIT Press, 1977).

[19] *Abstracts* (Honolulu: VI World Congress of Psychiatry, World Psychiatric Assn., 1977). The abstract of Freedman's article reads as follows:

To whom does the psychiatrist owe allegiance? This can be one of the most agonizing ethical problems confronting the psychiatrist. Role conflicts often confront the psychiatrist in day to day practice, but questions of allegiance can be particularly crucial to psychiatrists in universities, courts, prisons, the military, or governmental bodies. Does the psychiatrist owe primary allegiance to patient or employer? The latter may be private or governmental. If there is a contradiction between the patient's needs and the employer's demands, to whom does the psychiatrist owe first loyalty?

A further set of problems develops when information regarding a patient is requested. This may be a court order or simply a required duty. How far does confidentiality of communication extend? Who should have access to such communication and under what circumstances? There are other dilemmas facing the psychiatrist which vary from situation to situation, country to country, and culture to culture. The need for minimal international standards is of prime importance. The formulation of an internationally accepted code could be of immeasurable support to the psychiatrist confronted by unethical demands upon his services.

[20] Chalke's abstract reads: The need for specific guides to professionals, practicing in prisons, particularly psychiatrists, will be established. The grounds and principles that should underly such guidelines and the problems in reaching a national concensus are explored. Examples of some of the more controversial guidelines are described. The need for some world wide agreement on the conduct of psychiatrists working in the correctional field are established, and the various attempts to reach such agreement to date, outlined. The alternatives to enforce such conduct are explored.

and correctional psychiatry); Ehrhardt of Marburg and Bloomquist of Stock-holm,[21] presented papers on ethics in psychiatric practice; what is psychiatry and what is ethics.

The current issue of the *American Journal of Psychiatry* includes several papers relevant to ethics.[22] To what extent can professional ethics resolve the issues raised by Professor Robitscher?

A Methodology Towards Solutions

The Council of Ontario Universities' report on approaches in "Participatory Planning," although relating to universities, is worth examination.[23] The report says,

> Traditional methods of reaching decisions on matters affecting the public interest seem no longer adequate as the pace of change quickens. Perhaps they never were adequate; but as new technologies change our lives in often unpredictable ways, as society becomes more and more dependent on government for services, and as the demands on the public purse soar, more and more citizens and groups are pre-occupied as much with how decisions are made as with what the decisions are . . . This concern for the process of making decisions is evident in many of society's institutions. Its manifestations can be seen at the governmental level in the development of white papers and task force reports . . . it is evident that these are complex questions of great concern in relation to public policy and it is equally clear that finding answers is not the prerogative of any one group . . .
>
> Planning, in contrast, is not an act but a process which is charac-

---

[21] Bloomquist's abstract is as follows: To get a basis for discussion of the ethics of psychiatry I have tried to analyze the concepts "psychiatry" and "ethics" and to lay down normative definitions we can use for a world wide discussion of these issues at the present time. I have not been concerned about the "real" or correct meaning of these words, rather about their use today and what professionals as well as laypeople hold their denotations to be. My method has been a blend of empirical inquiry and literature research.

The inquiry shows both concepts to be used in a variety of ways, from very narrow to very broad, almost universal, denotations. "Psychiatry" can be used to mean anything between just the fraction of the medical science that deals with purely somatic diseases — brain tumors, Huntington's Chorea, etc. — which give mental symptoms, to the whole field of disturbances of interpersonal relationships. "Ethics," in a similar way, is sometimes defined as the study of a small fraction of language — propositions including words like good, bad, right, wrong, ought to etc. — but also the whole realm of human conduct. For our present purpose broad, but not universal definitions are recommended in an attempt to cover the different ethical issues the psychiatrists and the para-psychiatric staff meet in their everyday practice.

Further discussions will show whether or not we have to narrow our definitions and limit our tasks.

[22] *Am. J. Psychiat.* 135:2 (Feb. 1978). See R. A. Moore, "Ethics in the Practice of Psychiatry —Origins, Functions, Models, and Enforcement" at 157–163; P. G. Bourne, "The Psychiatrist's Responsibility and the Public Trust" at 174–177; J. Monahan, "Prediction Research and the Emergency Commitment of Dangerous Mentally Ill Persons: a Reconsideration" at 198–201; G. G. Affleck, M. A. Peszke, and R. M. Wintrob, "Psychiatrists' Familiarity with Legal Statutes Governing Emergency Involuntary Hospitalization" at 205–209.

[23] *Participatory Planning* Council of Ontario Universities Fifth Annual Review, 1970–71 (Toronto: Council of Ontario Universities, 1971).

terized by continuous adjustment. The higher the rate of change, the greater the need for planning . . . faster change means more difficult planning but makes a flexible planning and capacity to adjust plans to meet new realities all the more important. It requires acknowledging complexities, and involving interest groups with apparently conflicting goals. It involves too a process of learning. Participants cannot help but become sensitive to complexity and in doing so, become more judicious in their attitudes.

Are such principles sound to apply to the examination of psychiatric authority?

Currently, the following attempts to apply such principles are underway in Canada.

1. The Law Reform Commission of Canada has studied and submitted Reports to Parliament on many issues raised by Professor Robitscher. Reports entitled "Our Criminal Law," "Dispositions and Sentencing," "Mental Disorder in the Criminal Process," recommend changes in law on pre-trial issues, diversion, fitness, disposition, hospital orders, remands, etc., which are now under study by the Department of Justice. All are relevant in one way or another to psychiatric involvement and thereby authority.

The Commission is undertaking a new project, "Protection of Life" to evaluate present Canadian (federal) law protecting life and quality of life and to make proposals if necessary. This project is relevant to psychiatric authority with relationship to mutilation, sterilization, medical treatment of prisoners, informed consent, "treatment" in criminal law, personality and behavior control, chronic adult offenders, retarded offenders, alcoholics, drug addicts, sex offenders, and human experimentation.

2. The Royal Commission of Inquiry into the Confidentiality of Health Records under Mr. Justice Krever in Ontario will address itself to specific problems of psychiatric records, and possibly to psychiatric authority regarding release or withholding of clinical information, and patient/solicitor access to the patient's own medical record.

3. A third methodology is exemplified by the mandate given to the Ontario Council of Health by the Honorable D. Timbrell, Minister of Health, to undertake a Study on Mental Health Services in Ontario including a review of the Mental Health Act, the study under the chairmanship of Professor A. Lynch. There are four task forces — legal, primary services, specialized services, and maintenance and rehabilitation. Such an undertaking unquestionably will review study, receive submissions, and make recommendations pertaining to psychiatric authority.

Certainly, these various undertakings suggest that this is indeed an appropriate time" . . . to think about and to set limits for (or at least to scrupulously examine) the exercise of authority." As Professor Robitscher continues, " . . . many of the determinations made by psychiatrists need to be made by someone in society. . . . " Who shall it be?